This book belongs to

....

....

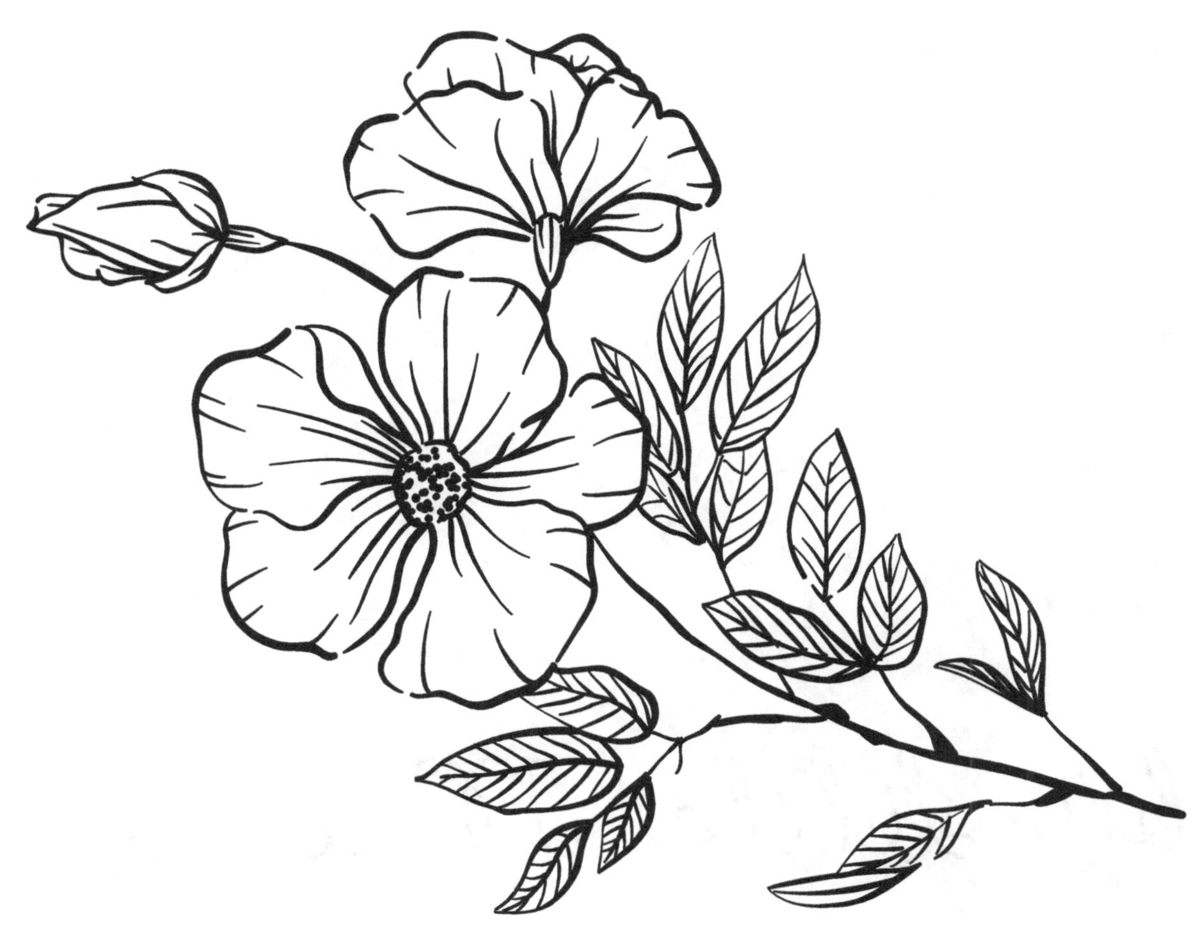

COLORING BOOK

by Little Mary

COLORING BOOK

by Little Mary

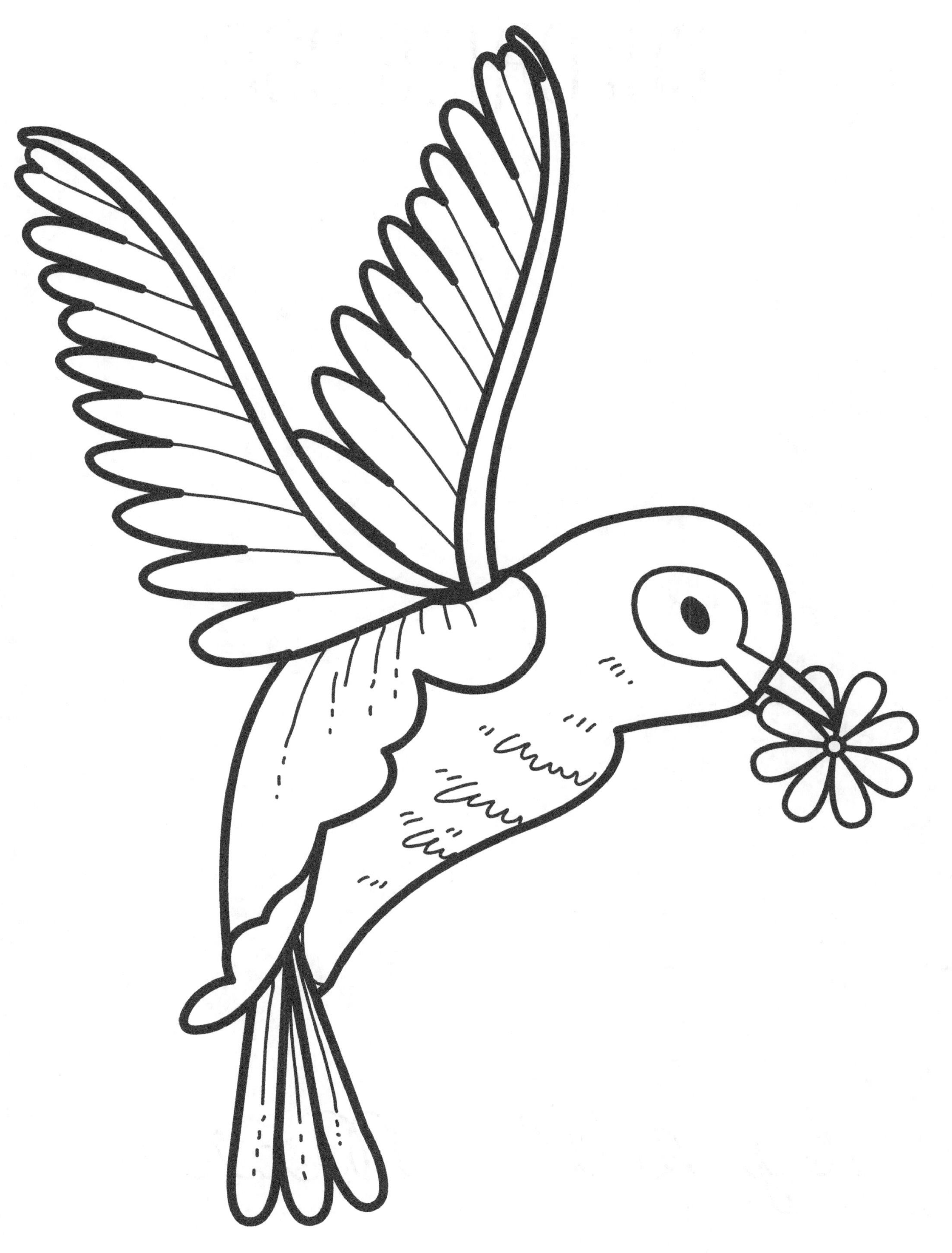

COLORING BOOK

by Little Mary

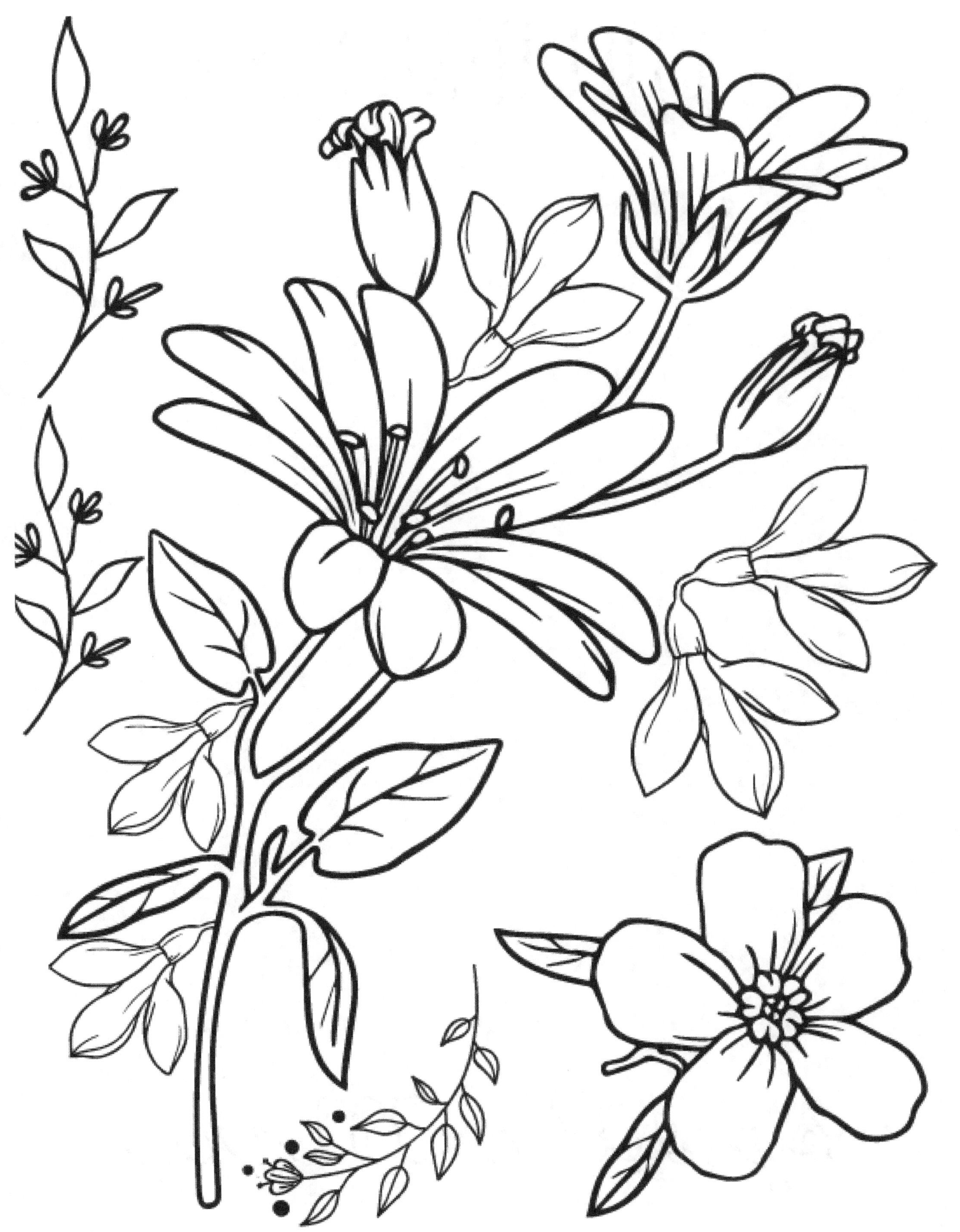

COLORING BOOK

by Little Mary

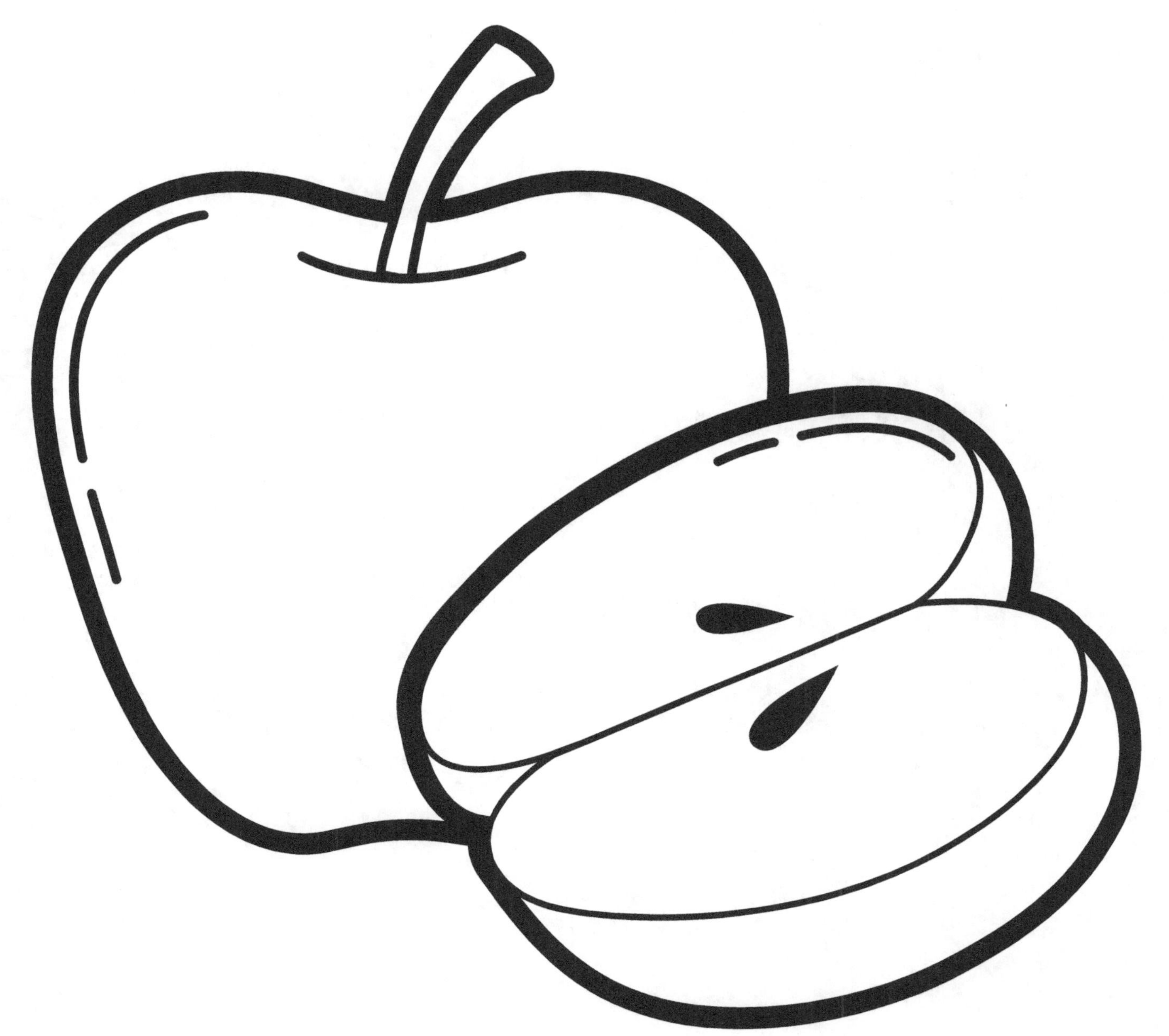

COLORING BOOK

by Little Mary

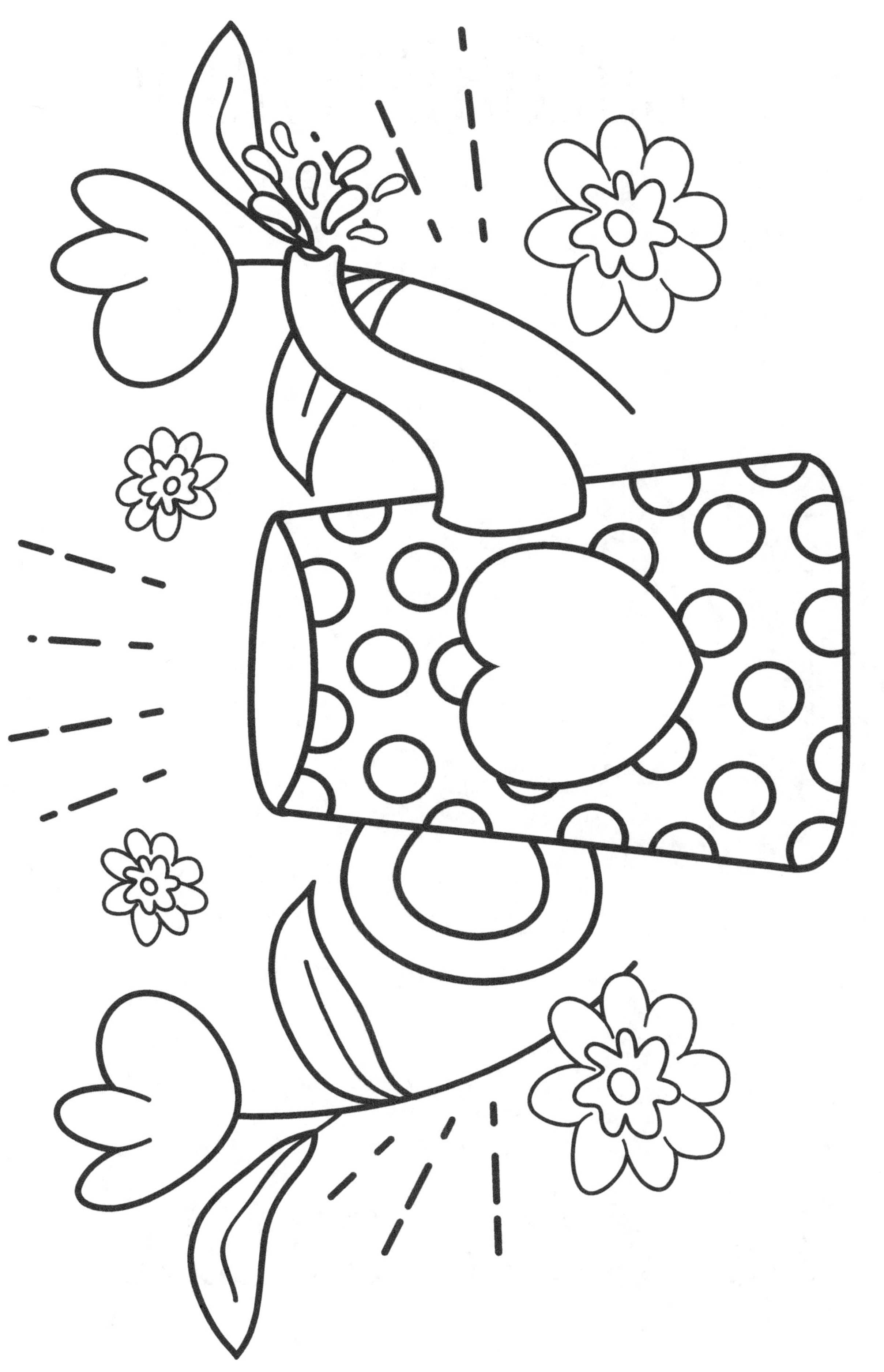

COLORING BOOK

by Little Mary

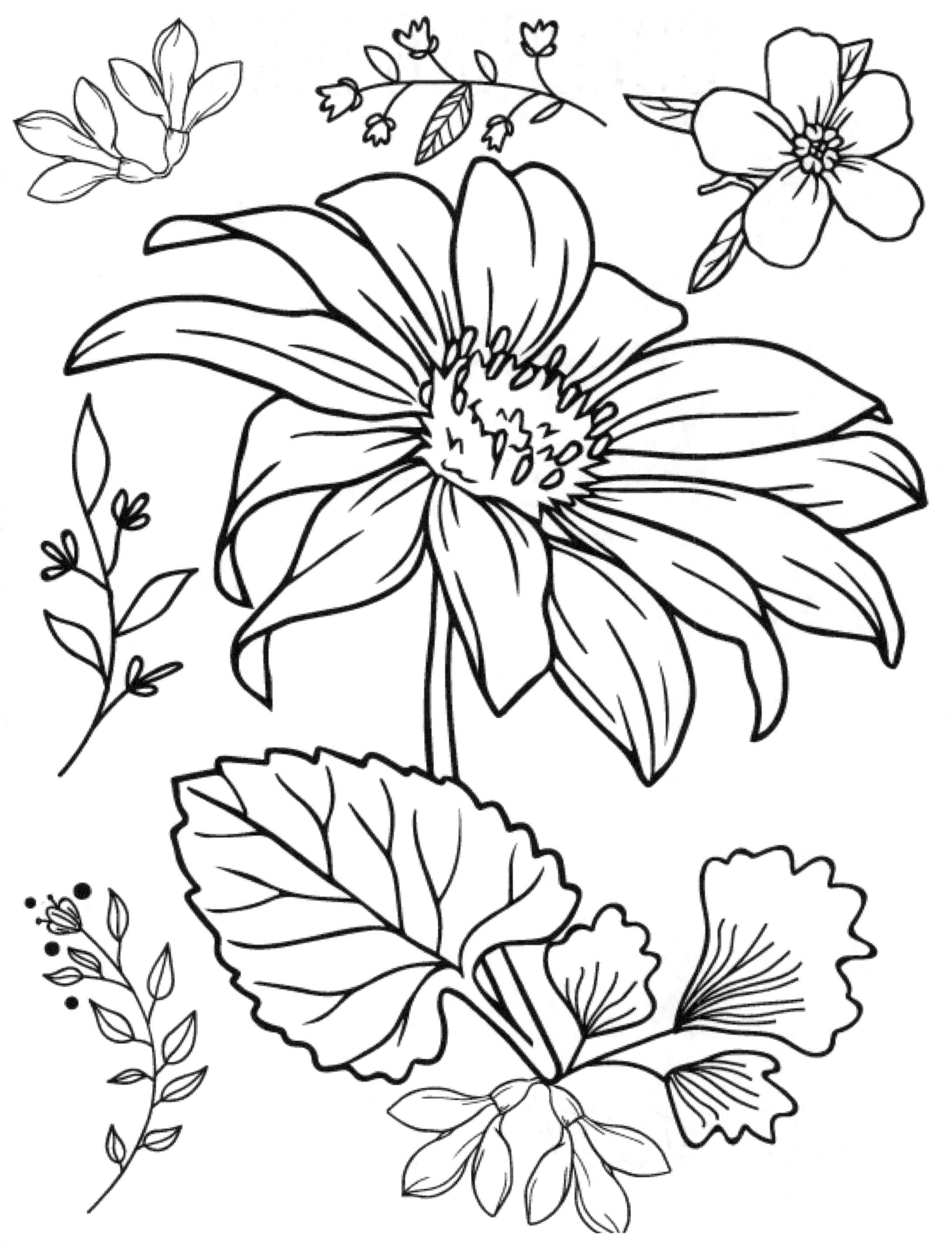

COLORING BOOK

by Little Mary

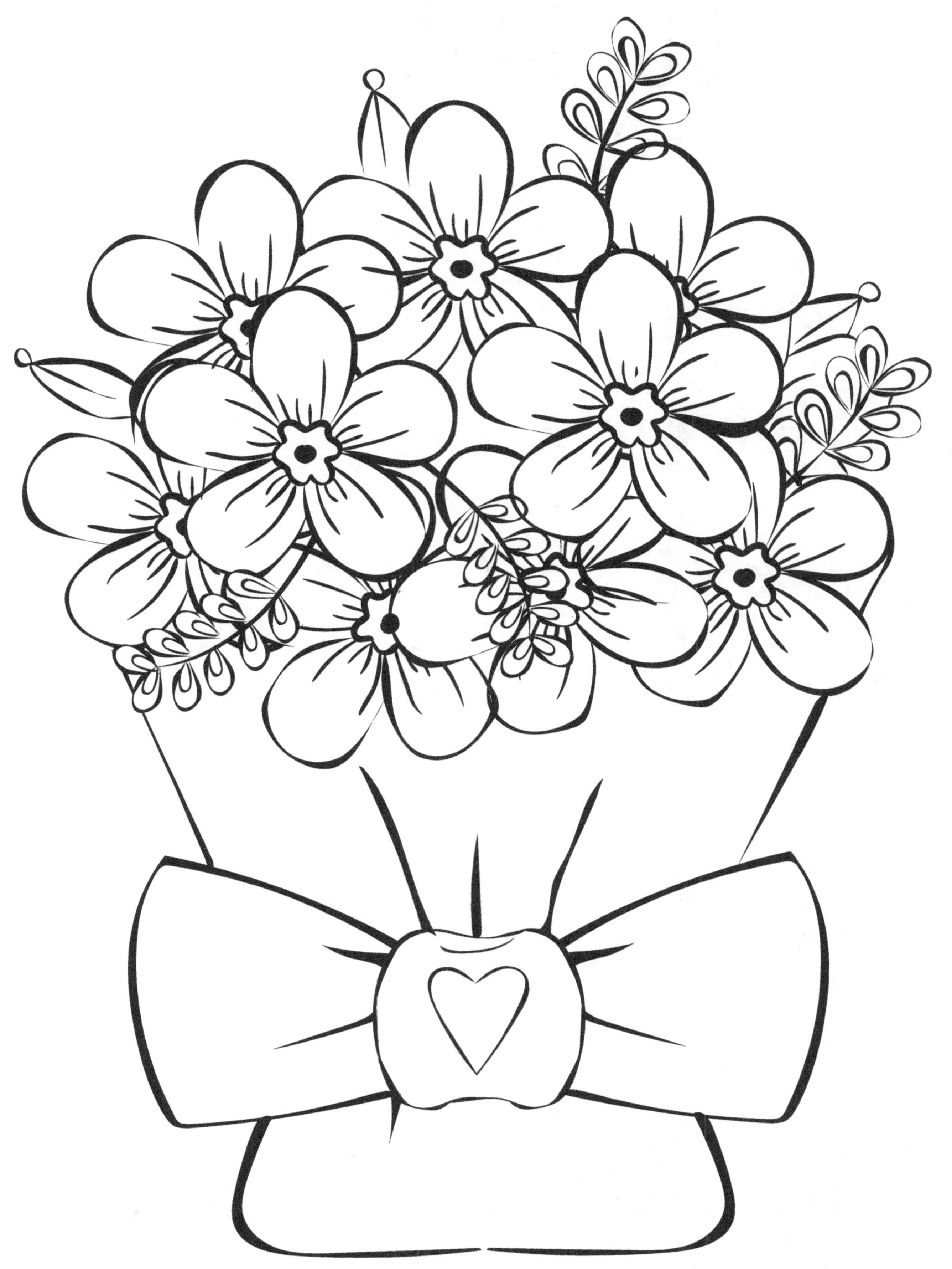

COLORING BOOK

by Little Mary

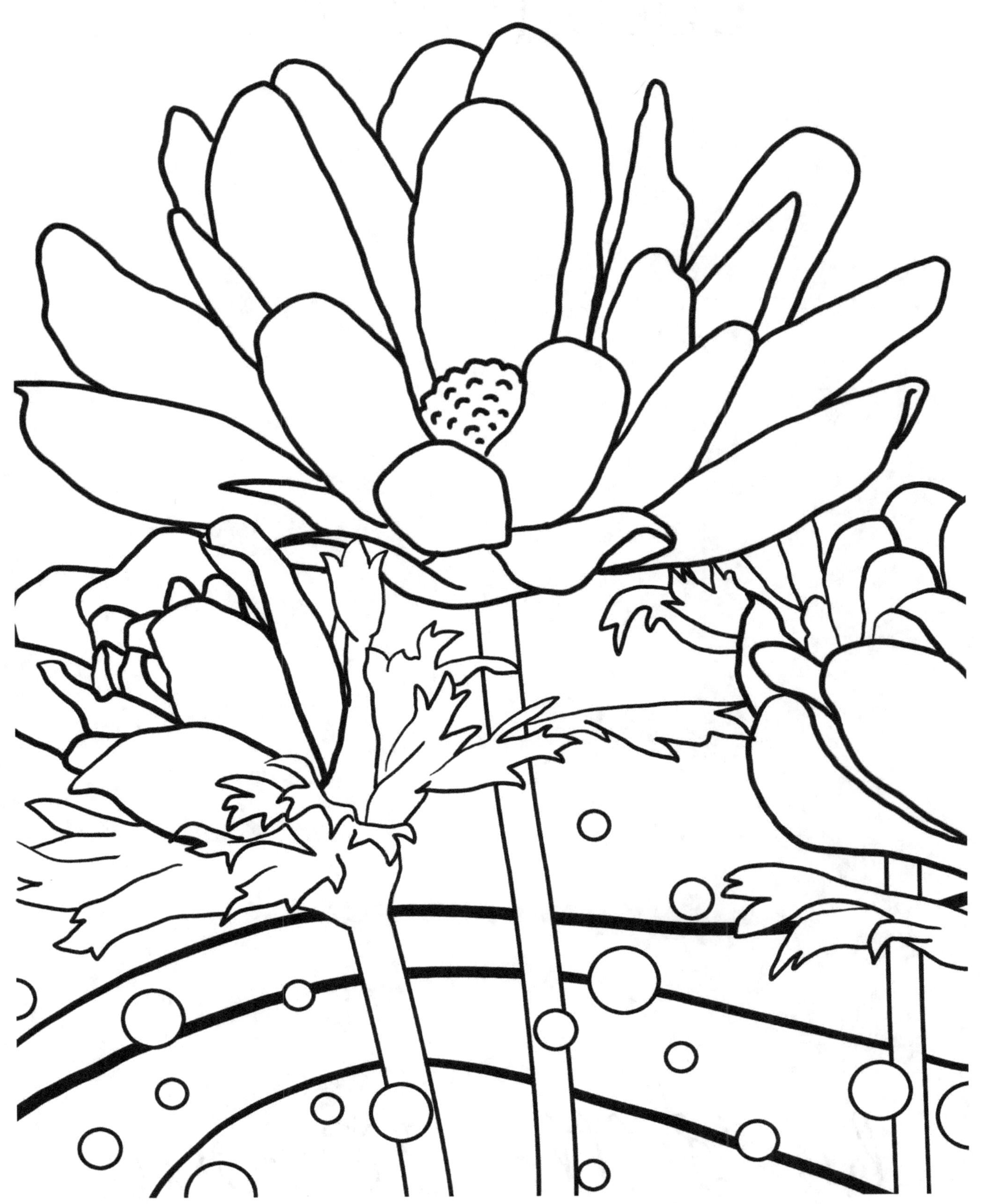

COLORING BOOK

by Little Mary

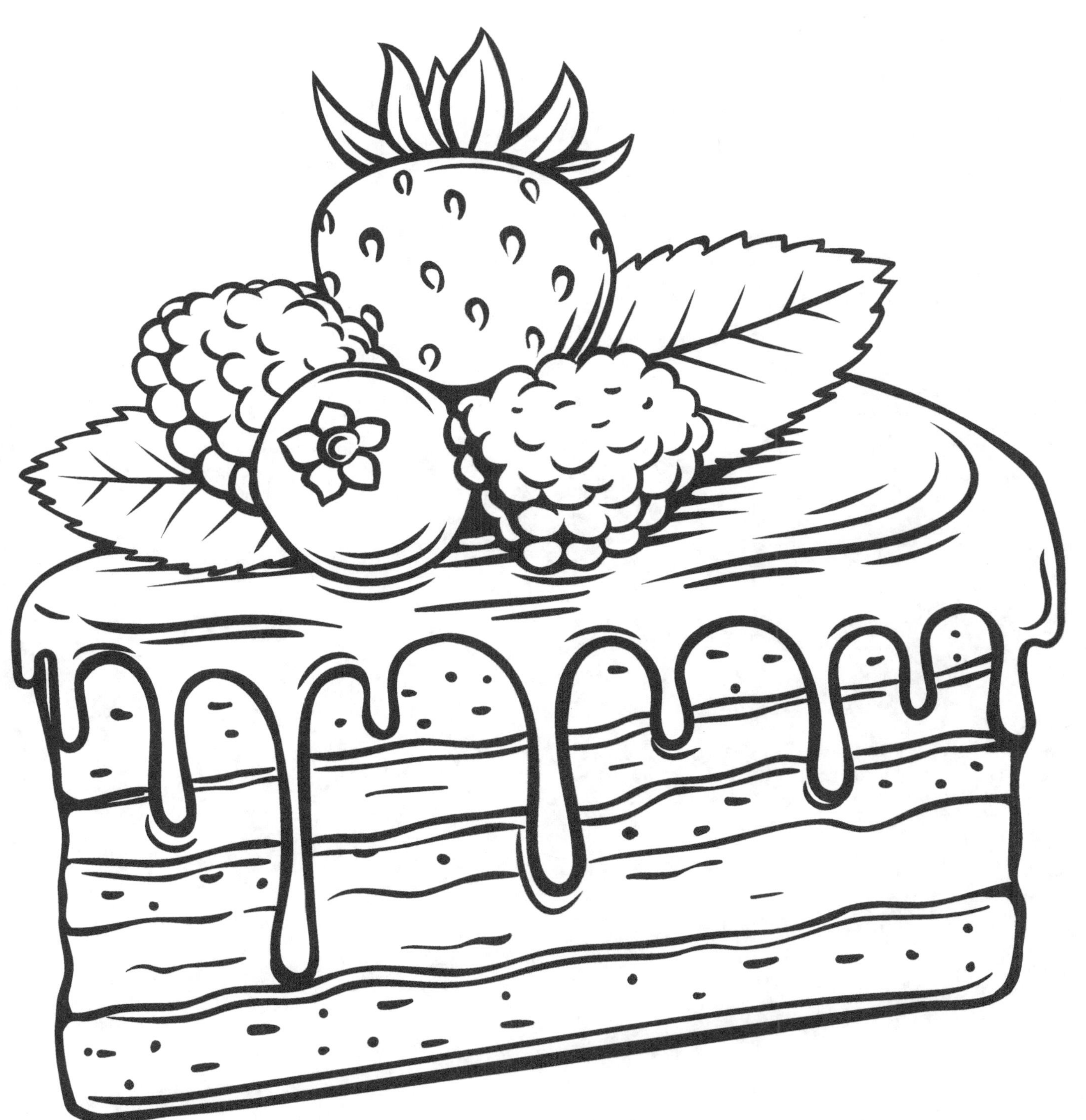

COLORING BOOK

by Little Mary

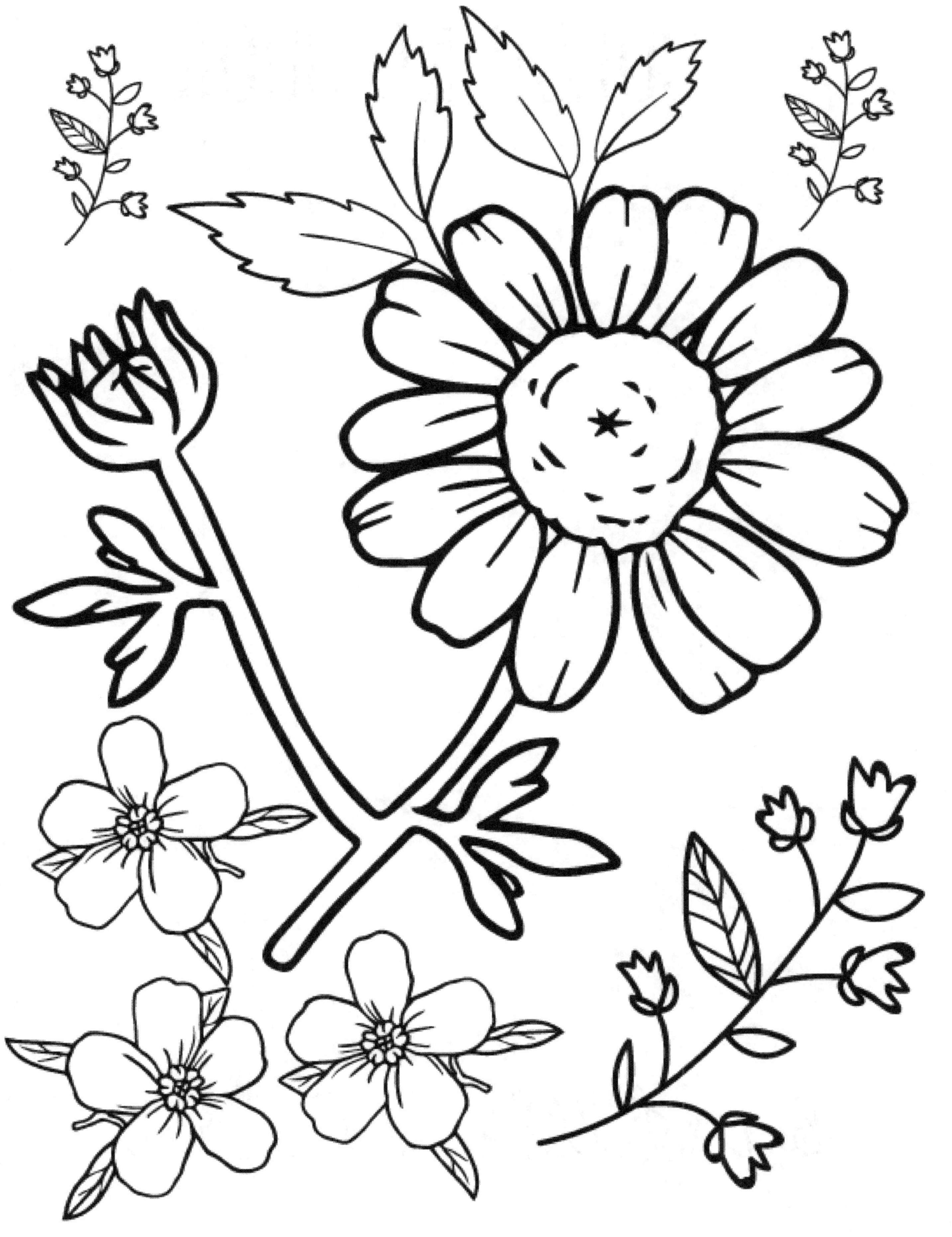

COLORING BOOK

by Little Mary

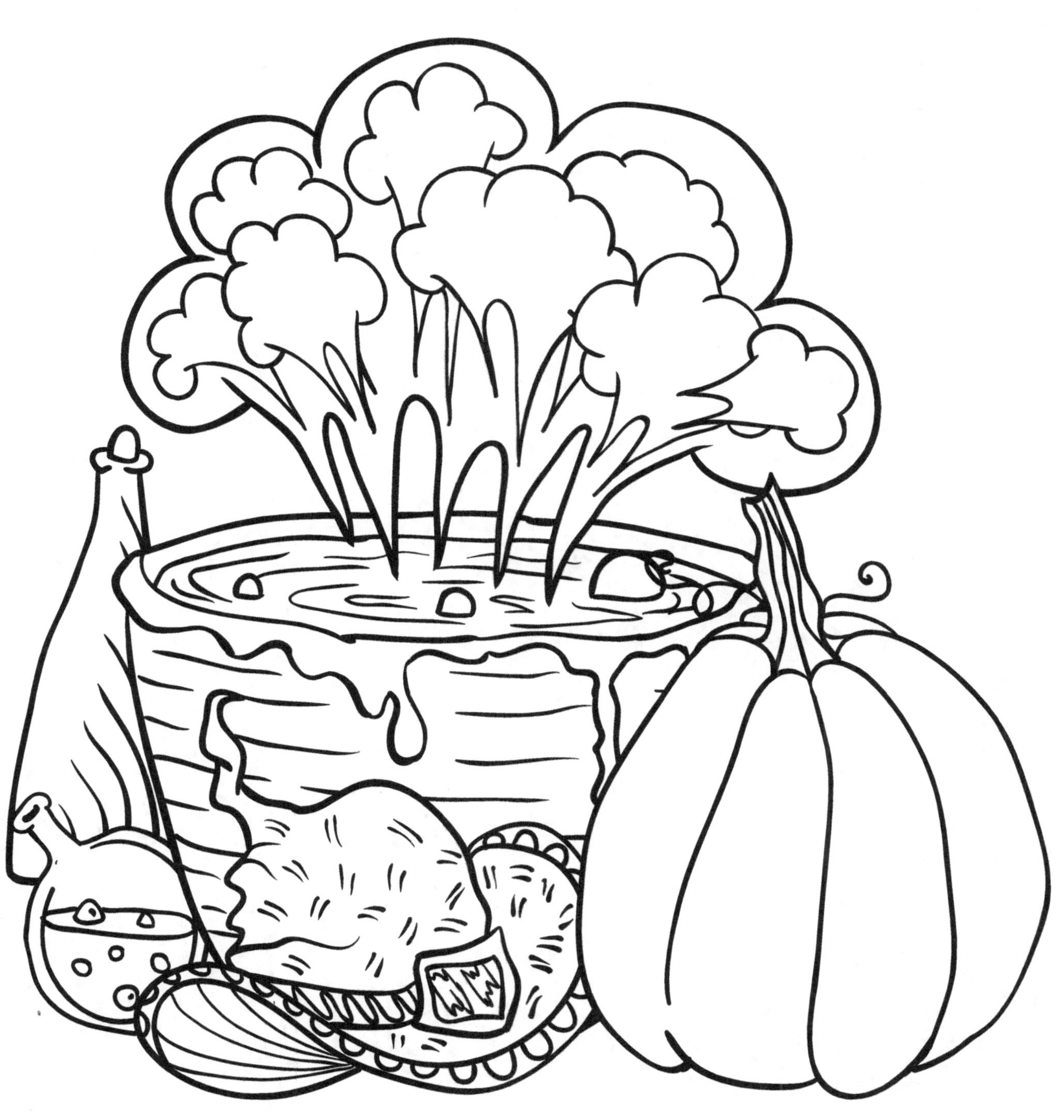

COLORING BOOK

by Little Mary

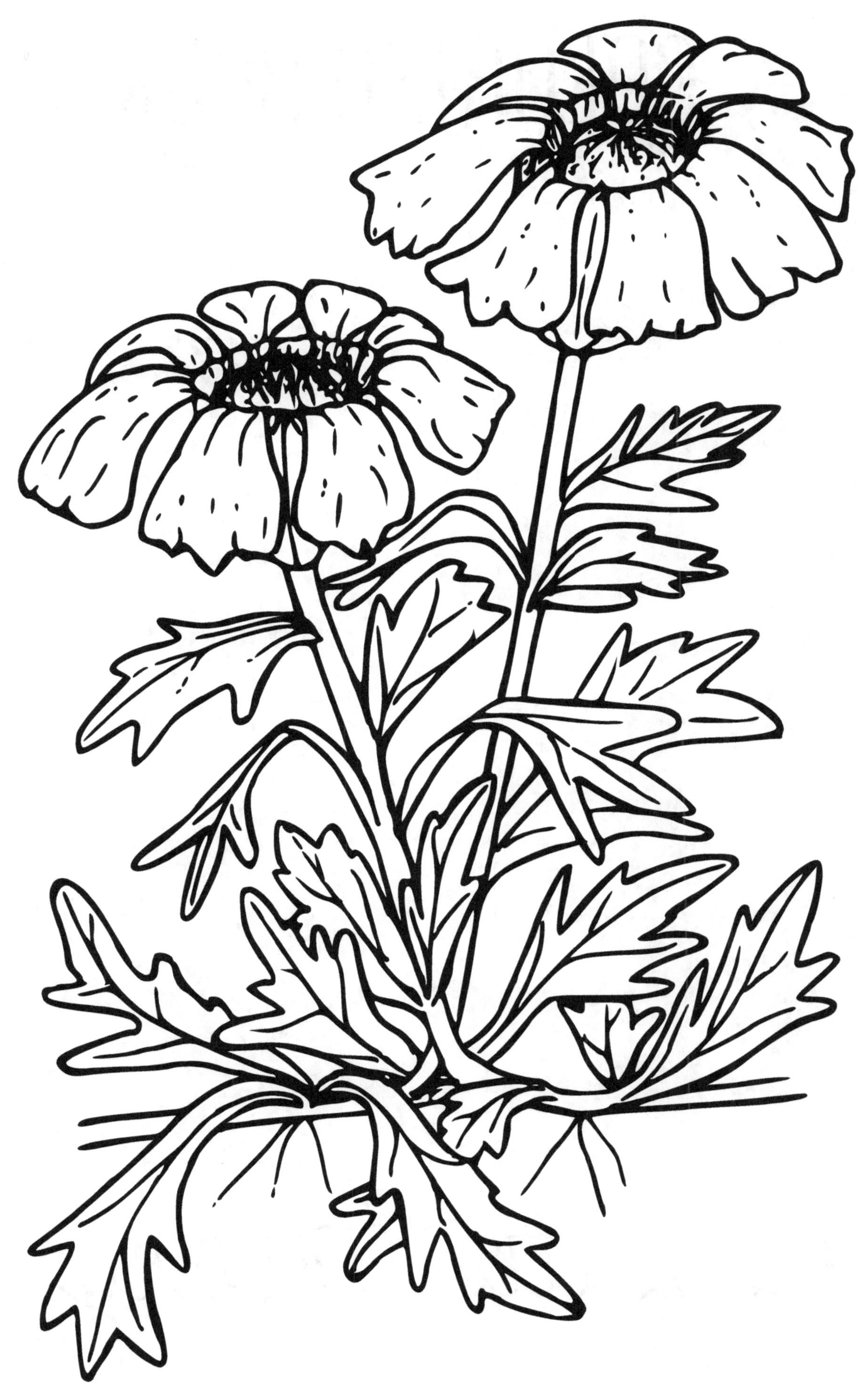

COLORING BOOK

by Little Mary

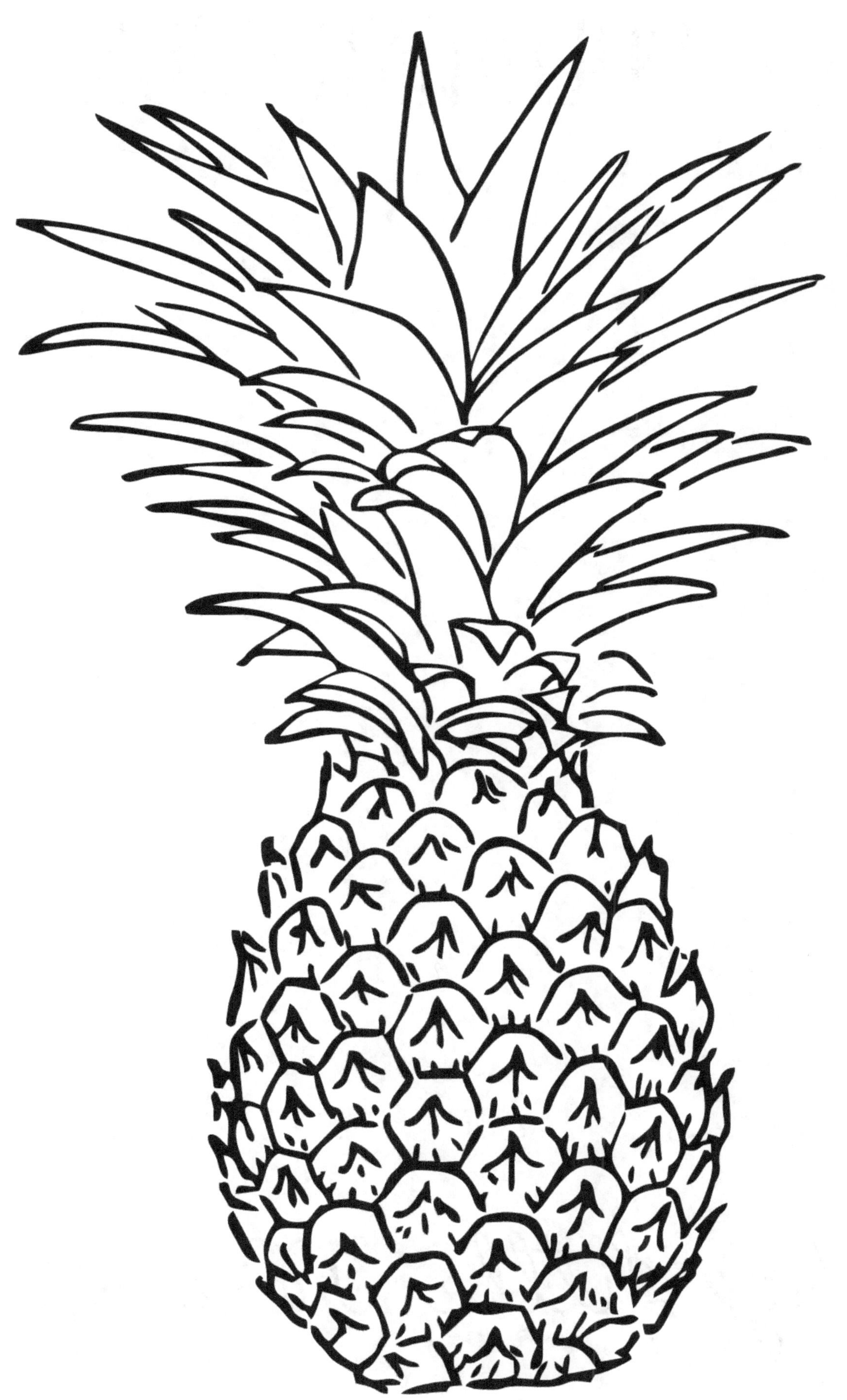

COLORING BOOK

by Little Mary

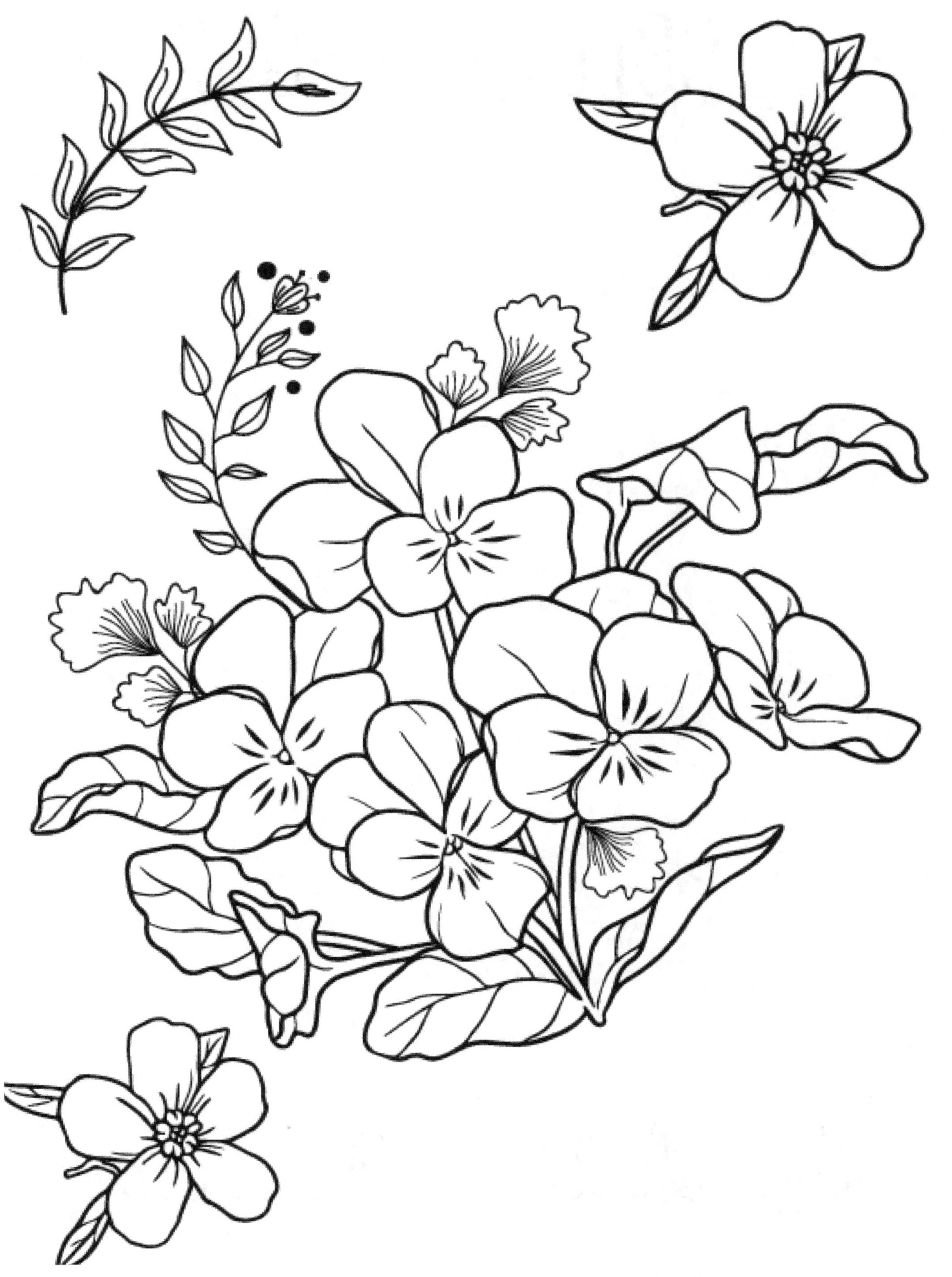

COLORING BOOK

by Little Mary

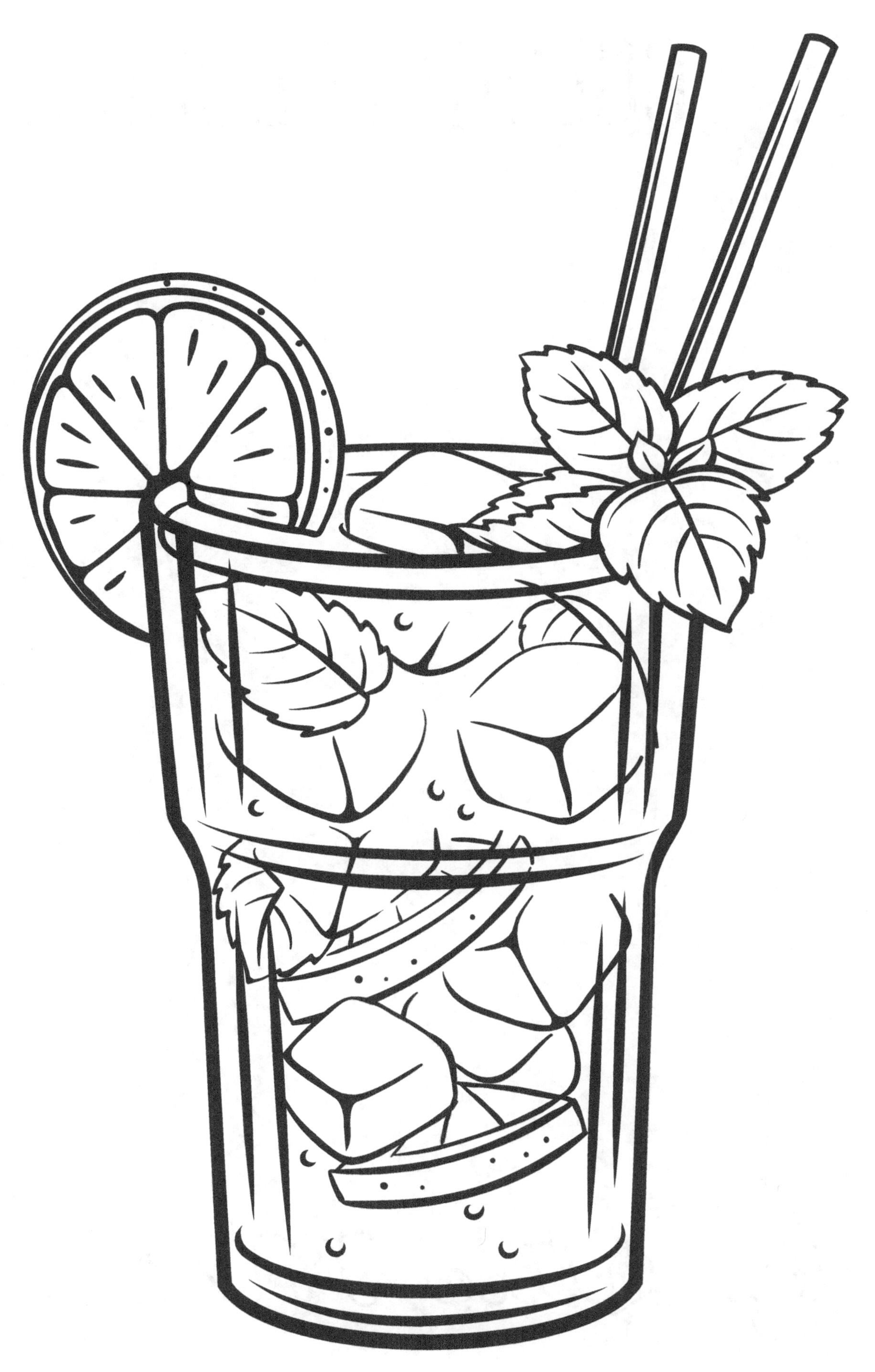

COLORING BOOK

by Little Mary

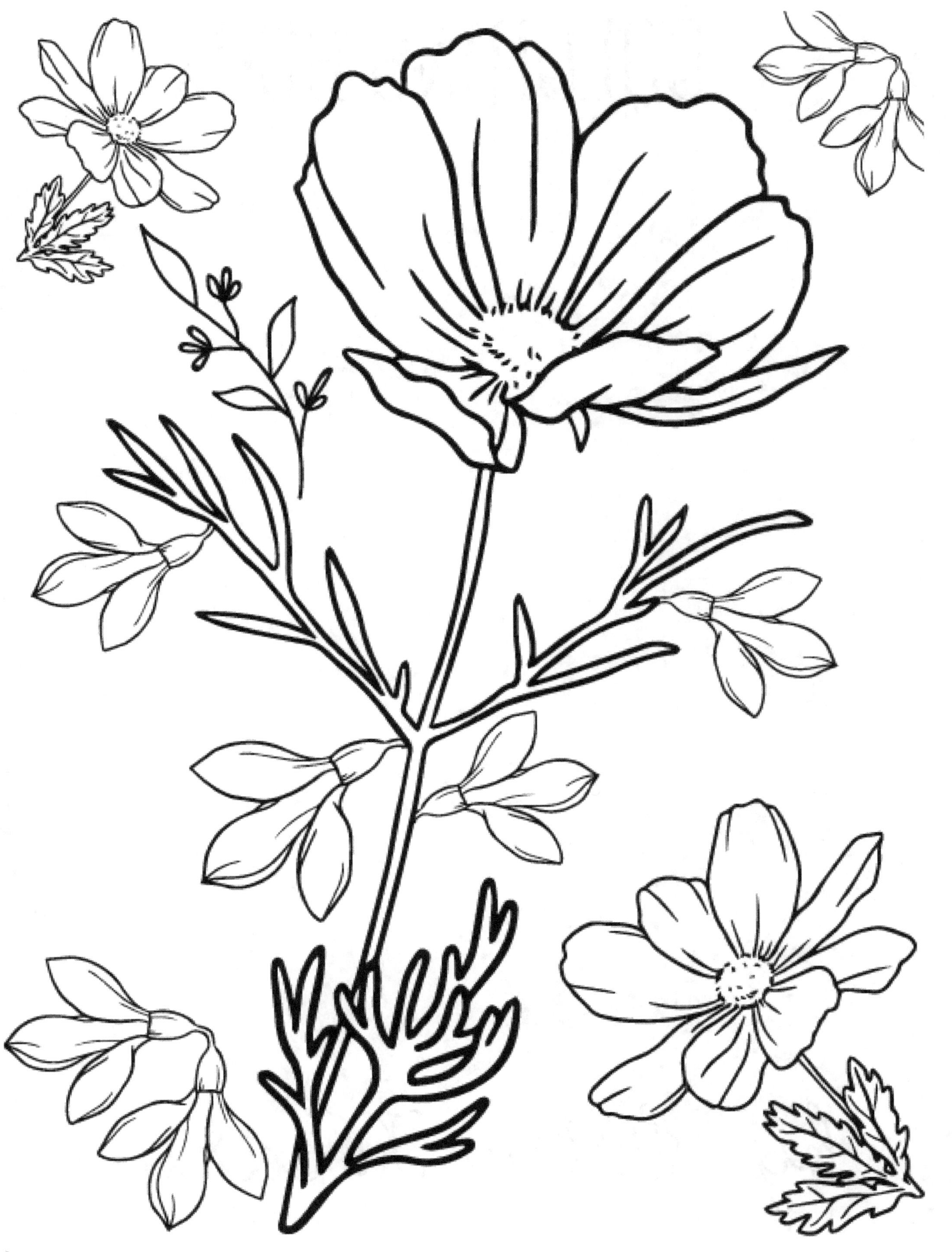

COLORING BOOK

by Little Mary

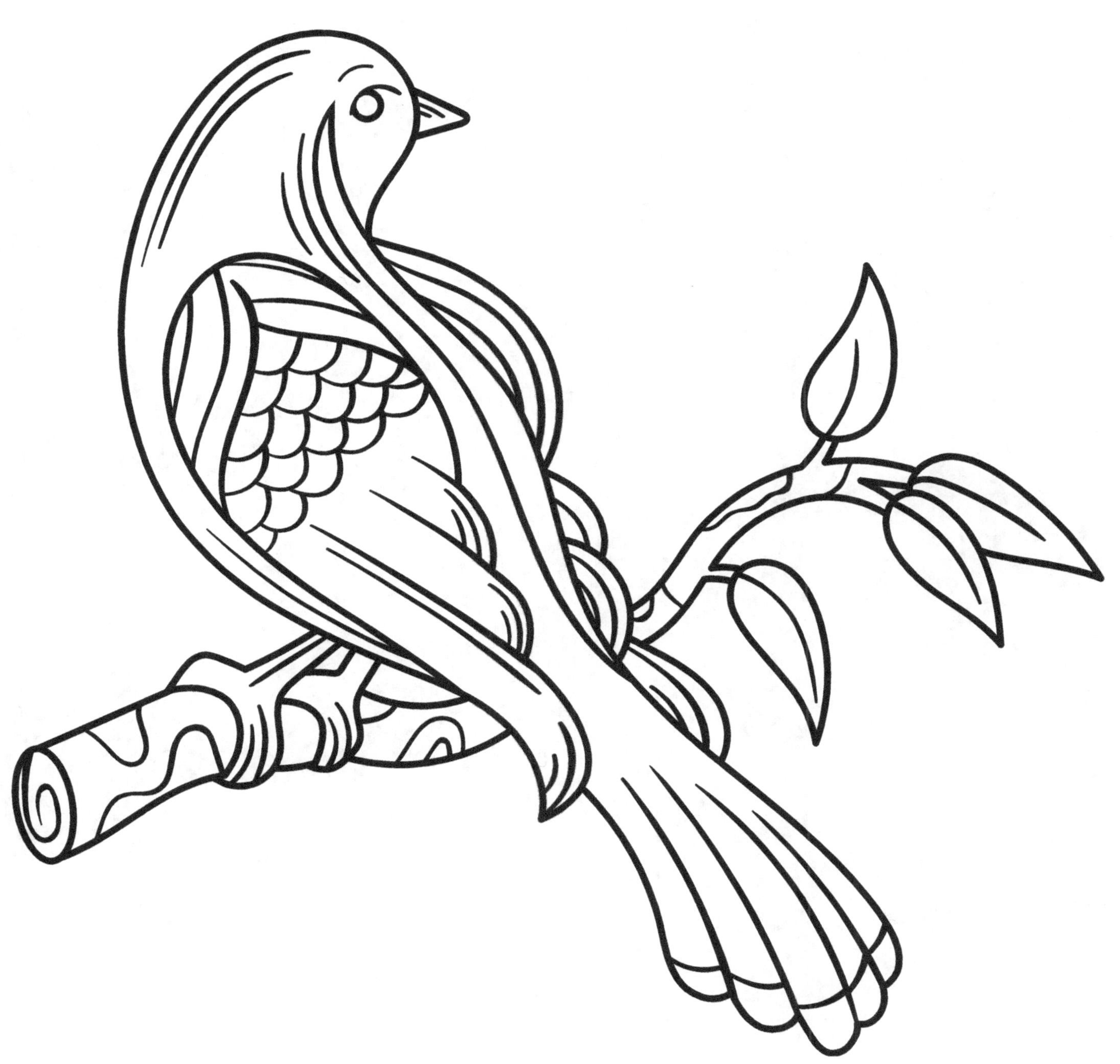

COLORING BOOK

by Little Mary

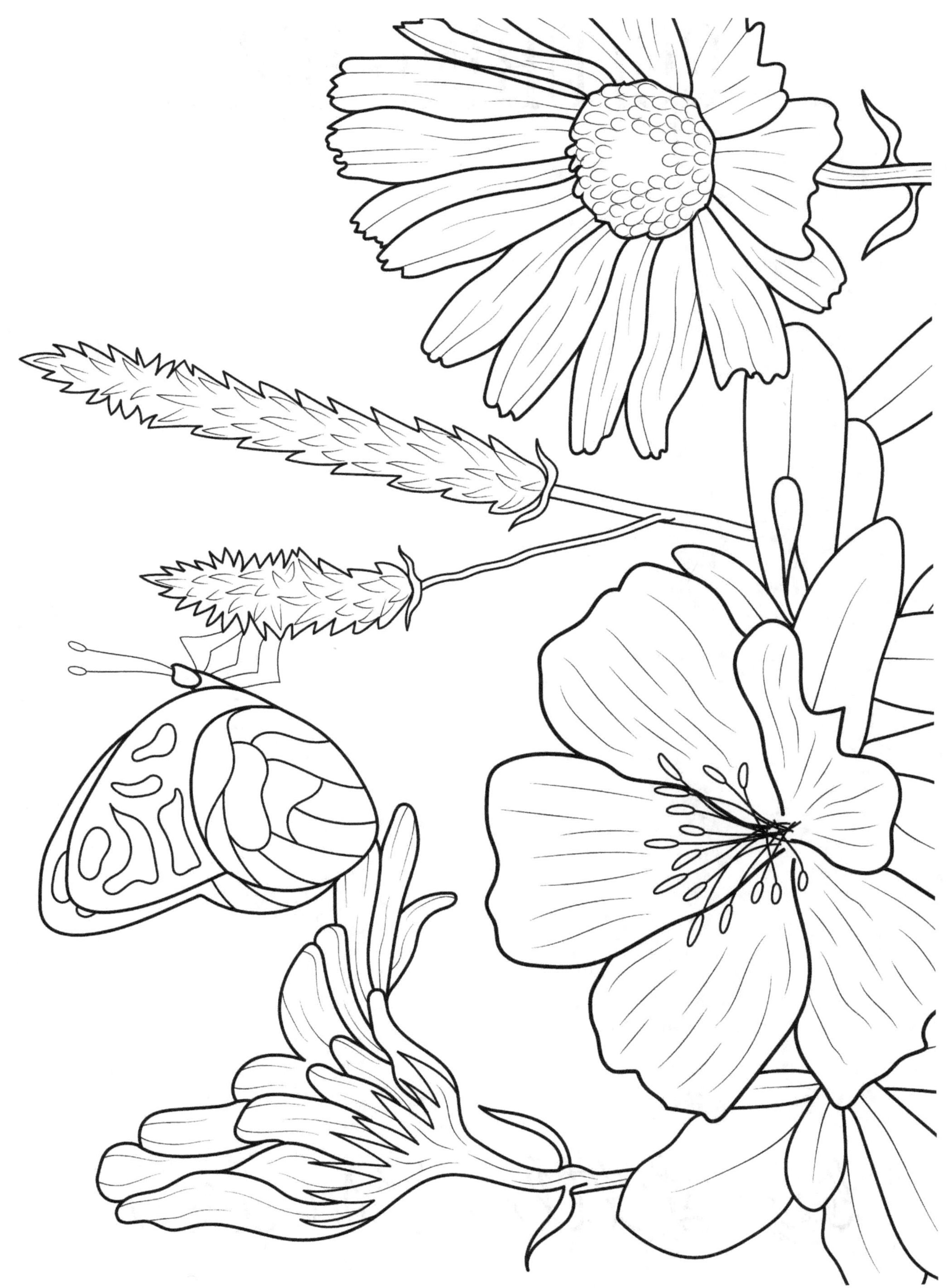

COLORING BOOK

by Little Mary

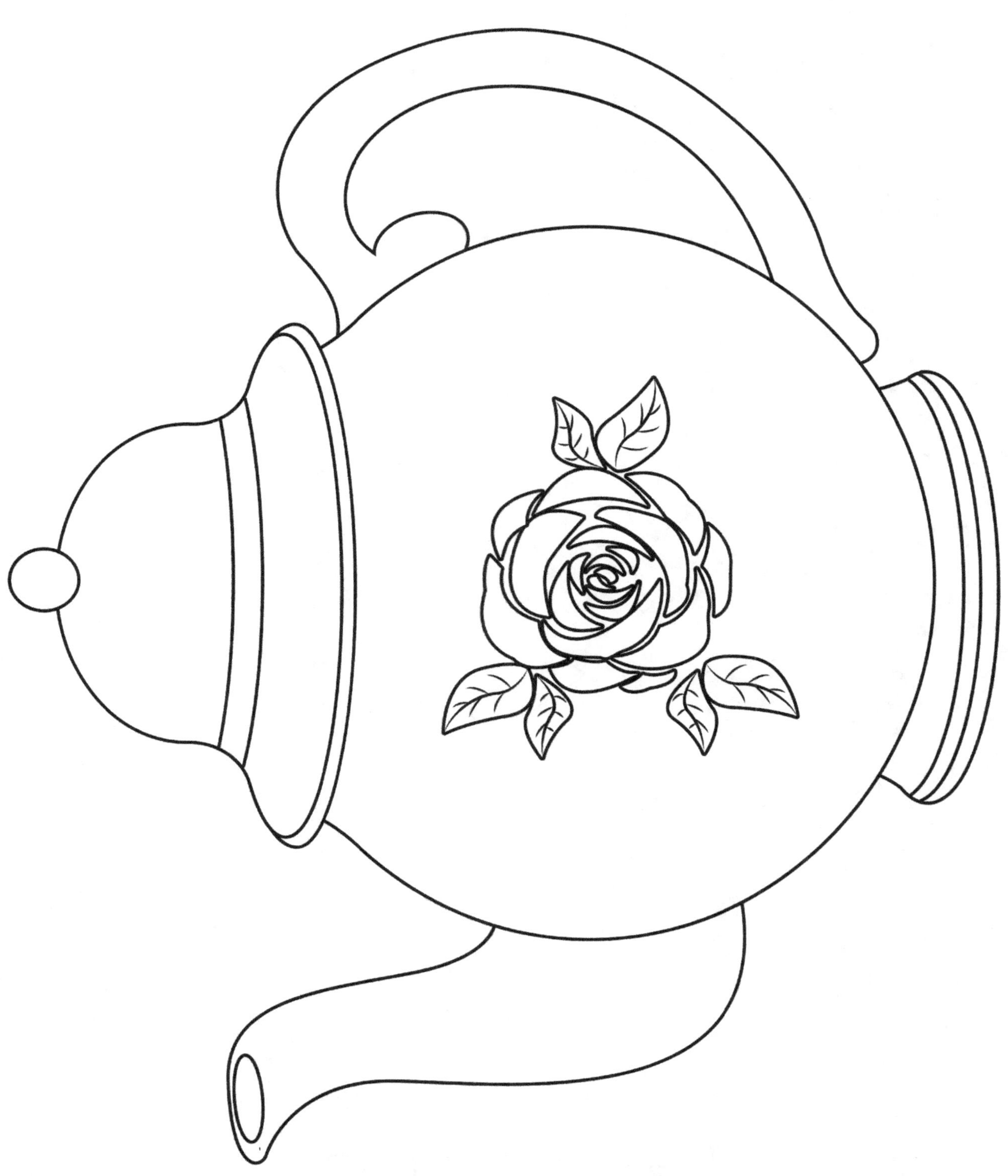

COLORING BOOK

by Little Mary

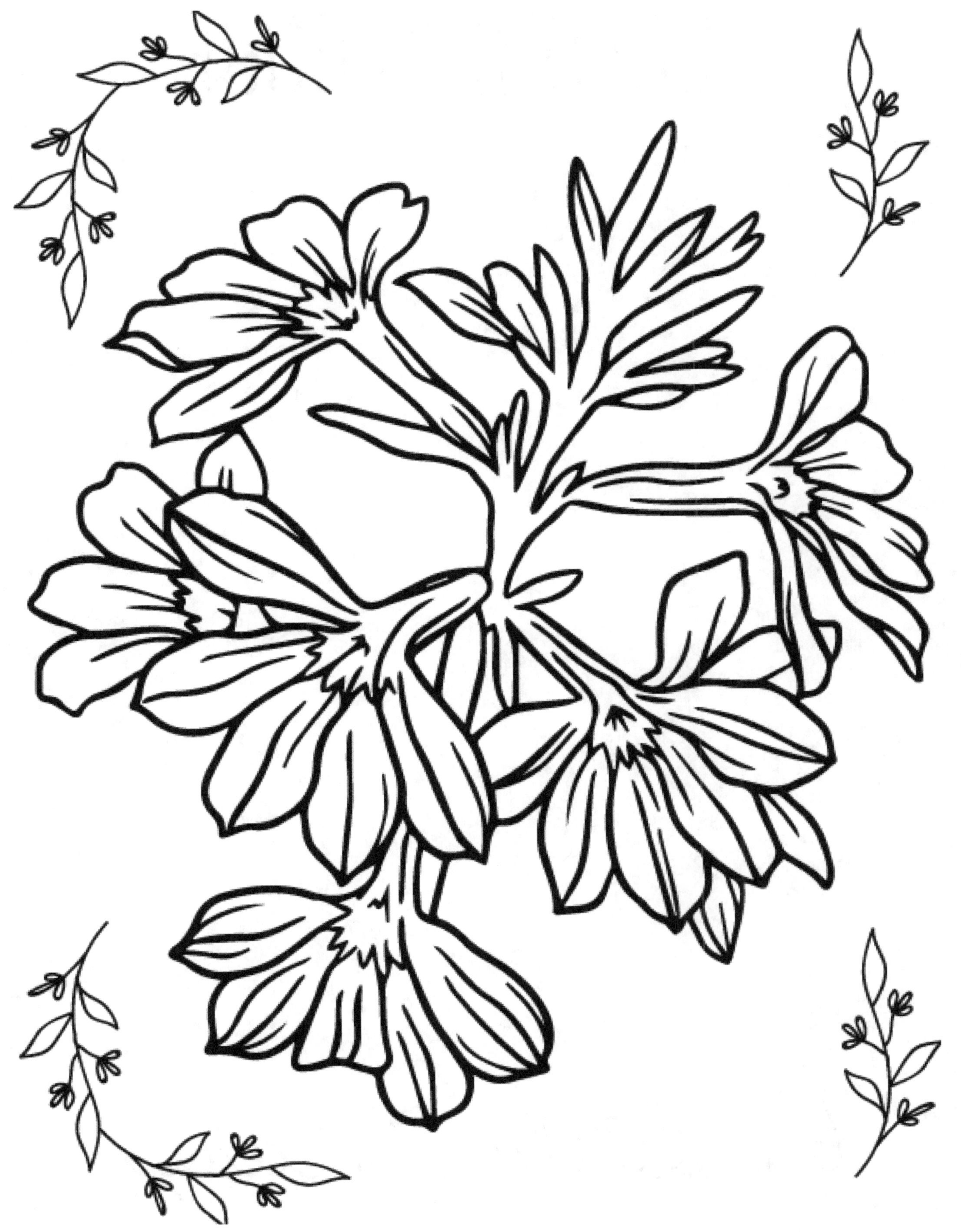

COLORING BOOK

by Little Mary

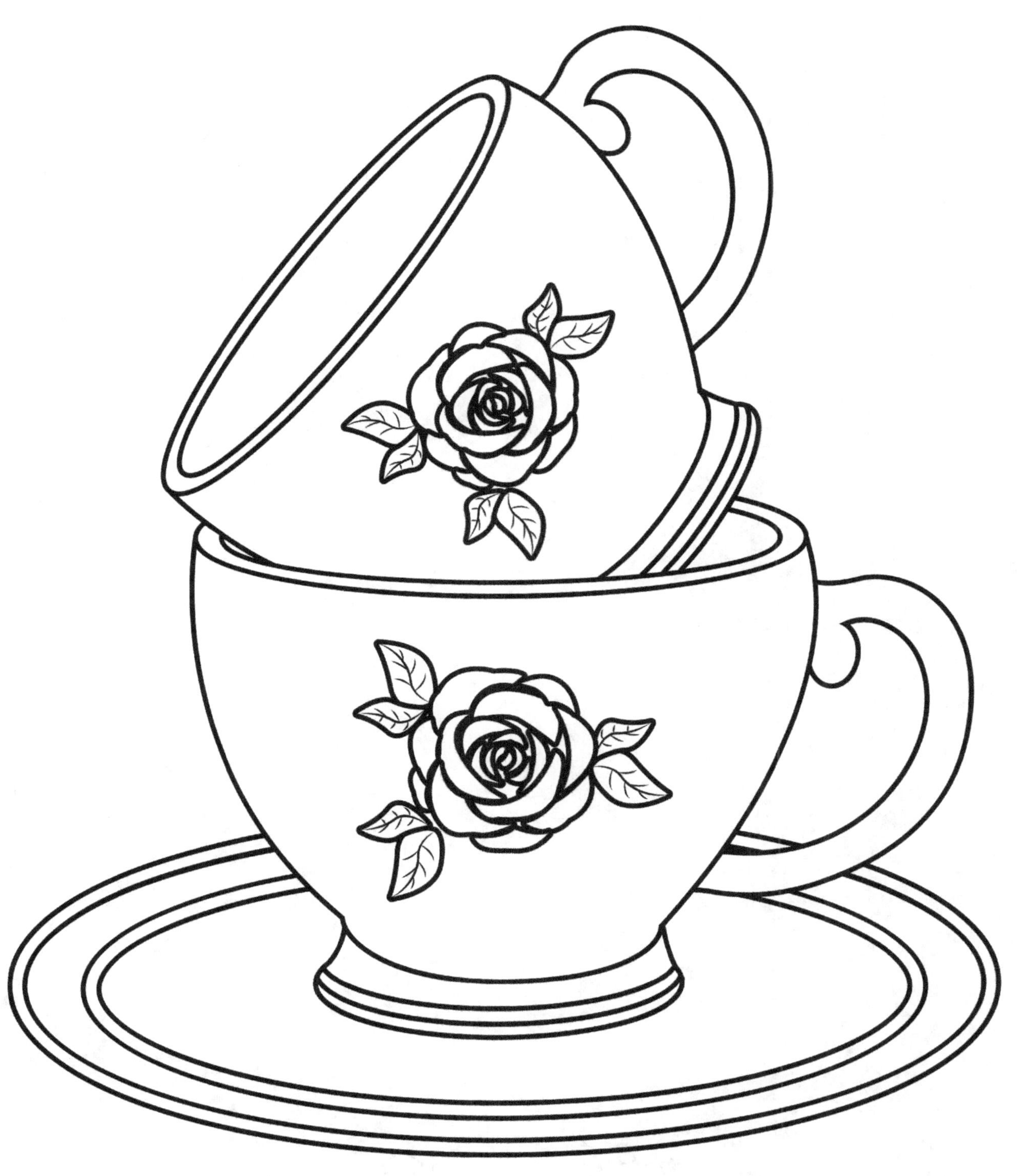

COLORING BOOK

by Little Mary

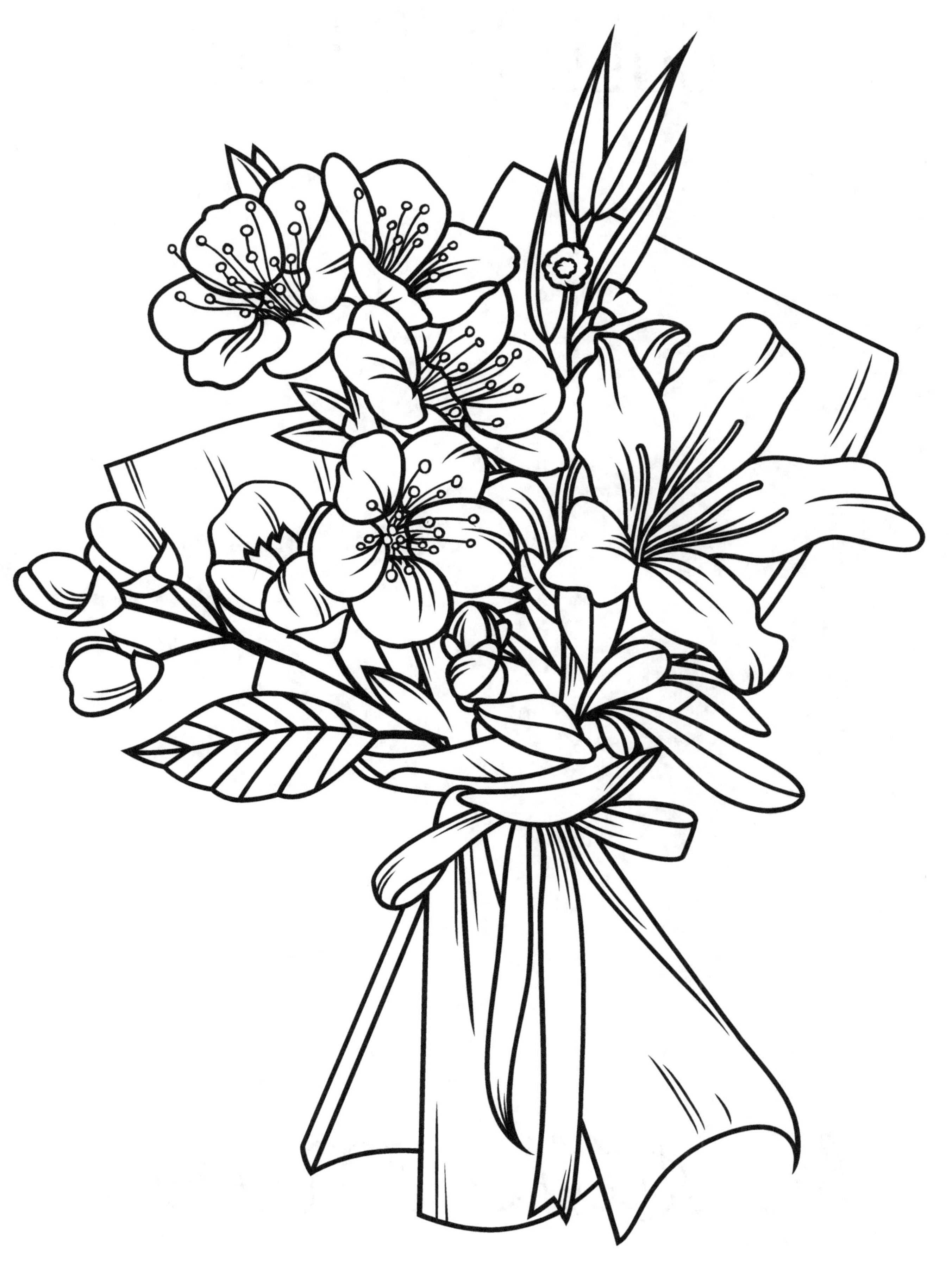

COLORING BOOK

by Little Mary

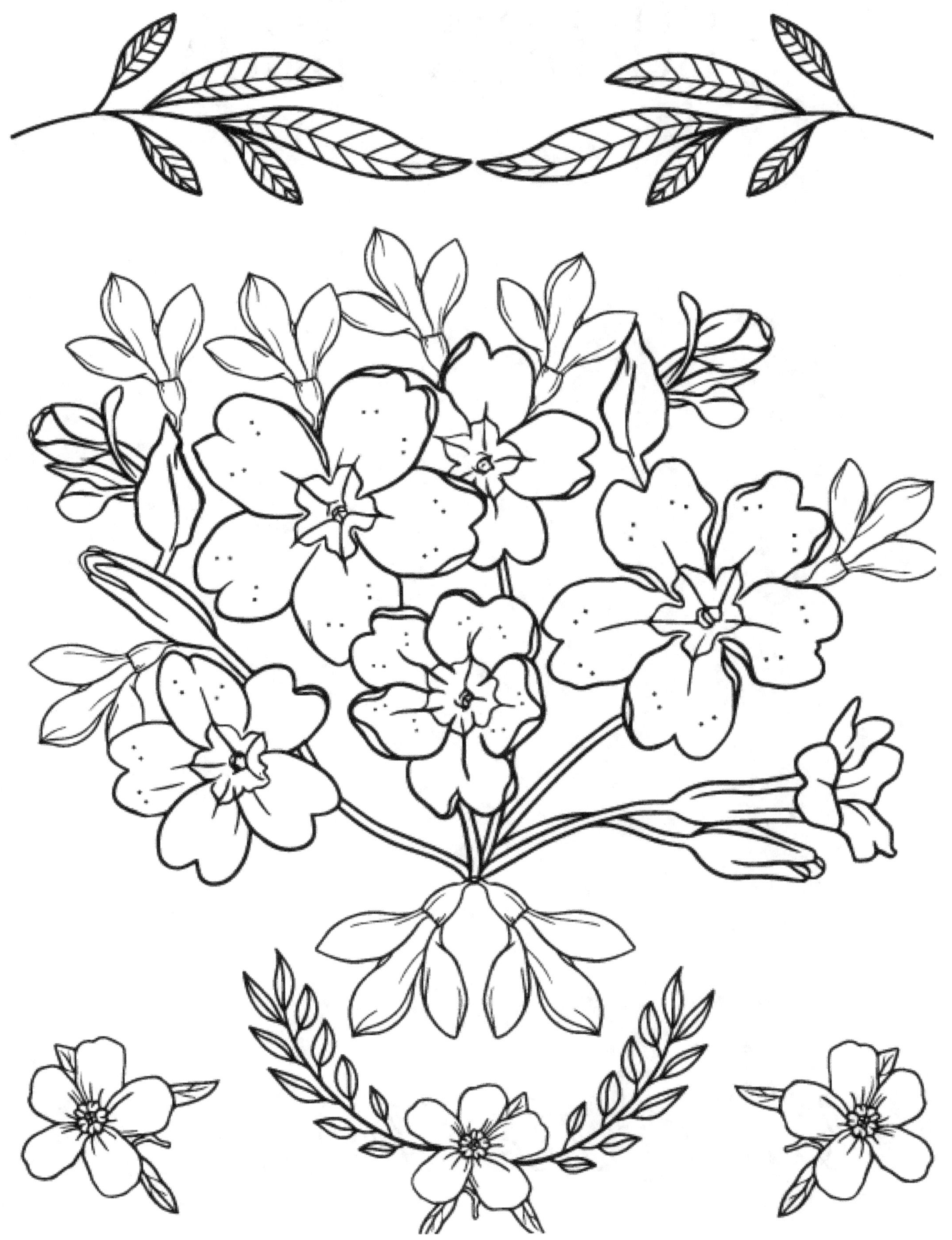

COLORING BOOK

by Little Mary

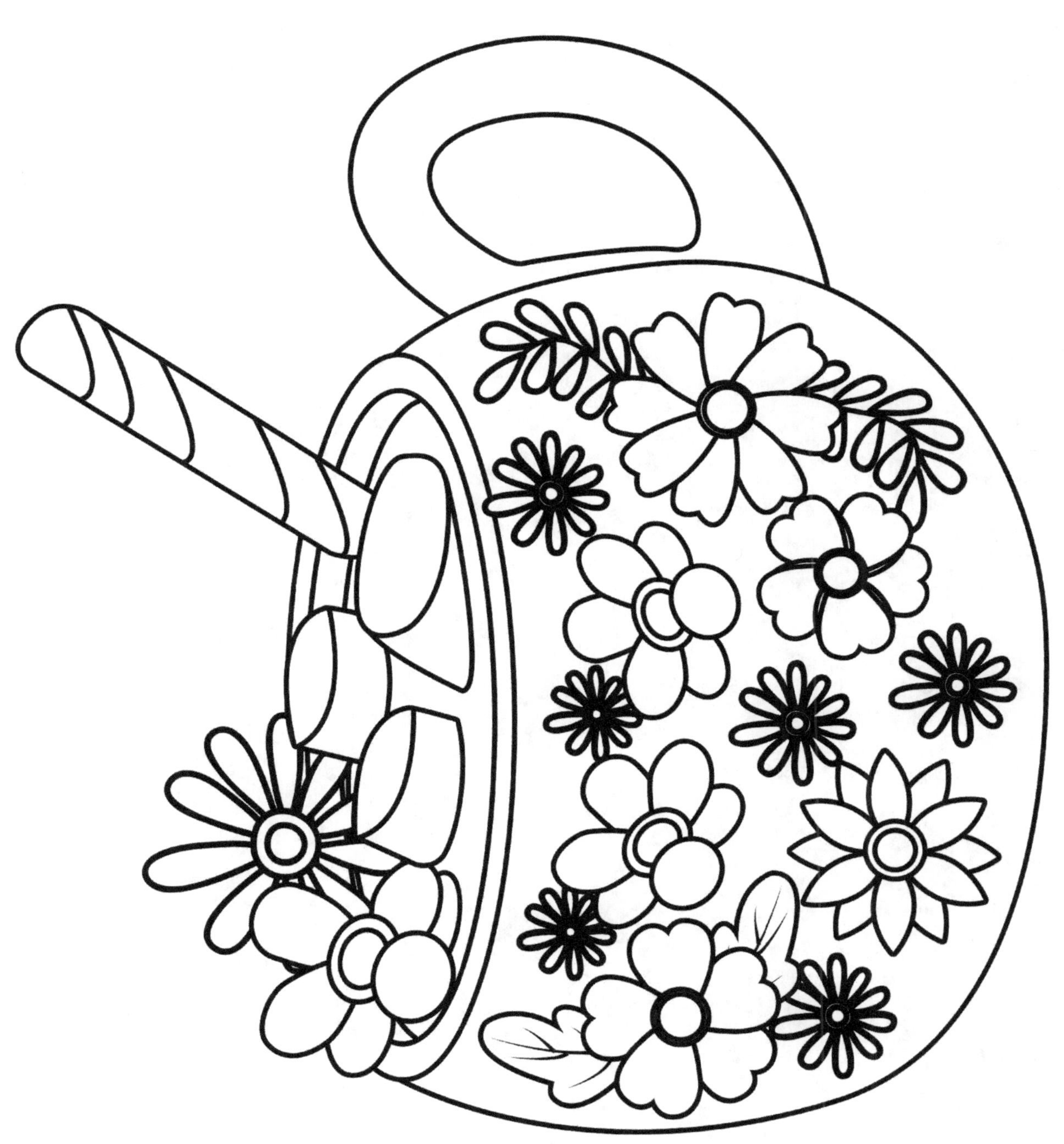

COLORING BOOK

by Little Mary

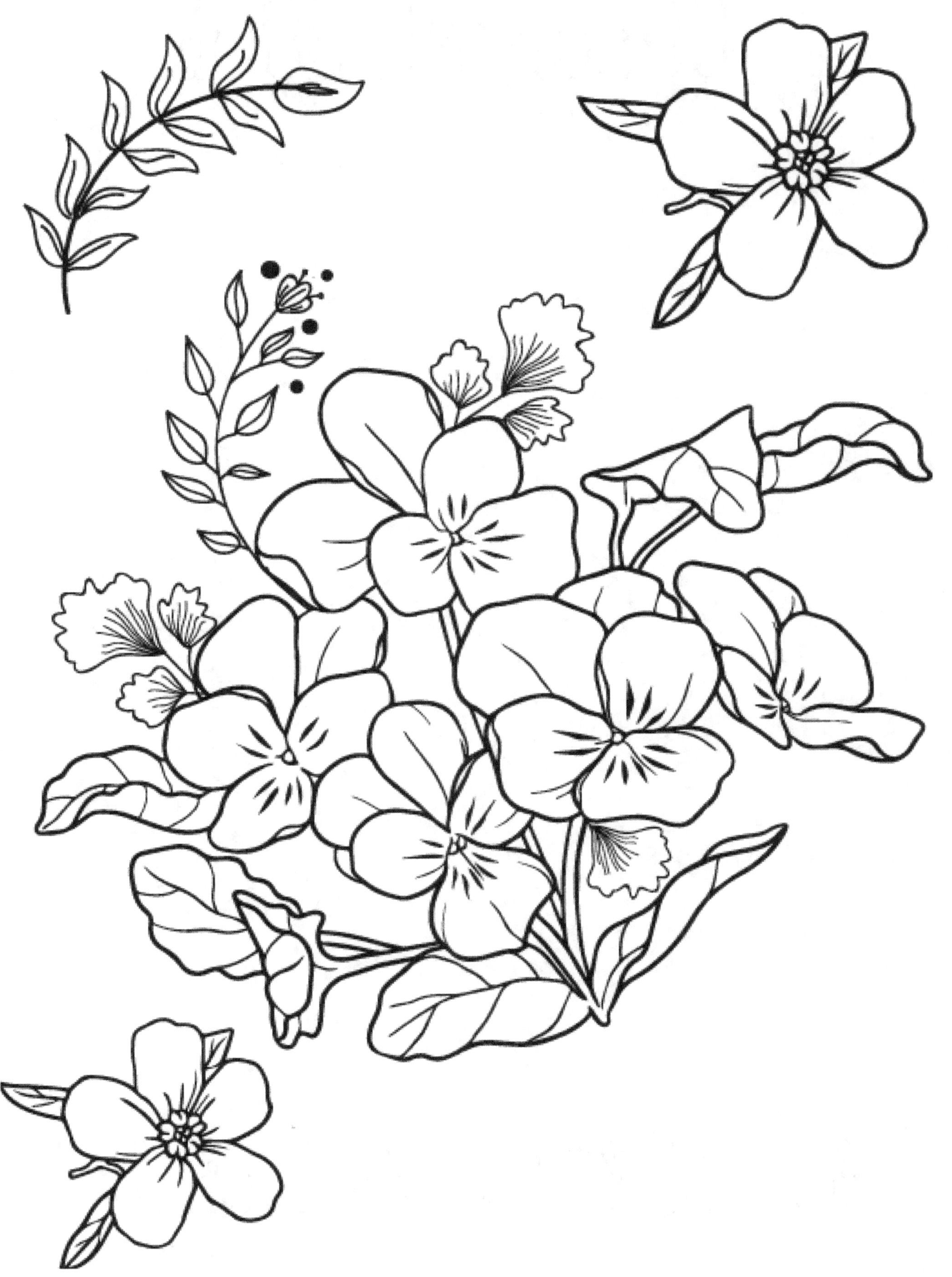

COLORING BOOK

by Little Mary

COLORING BOOK

by Little Mary

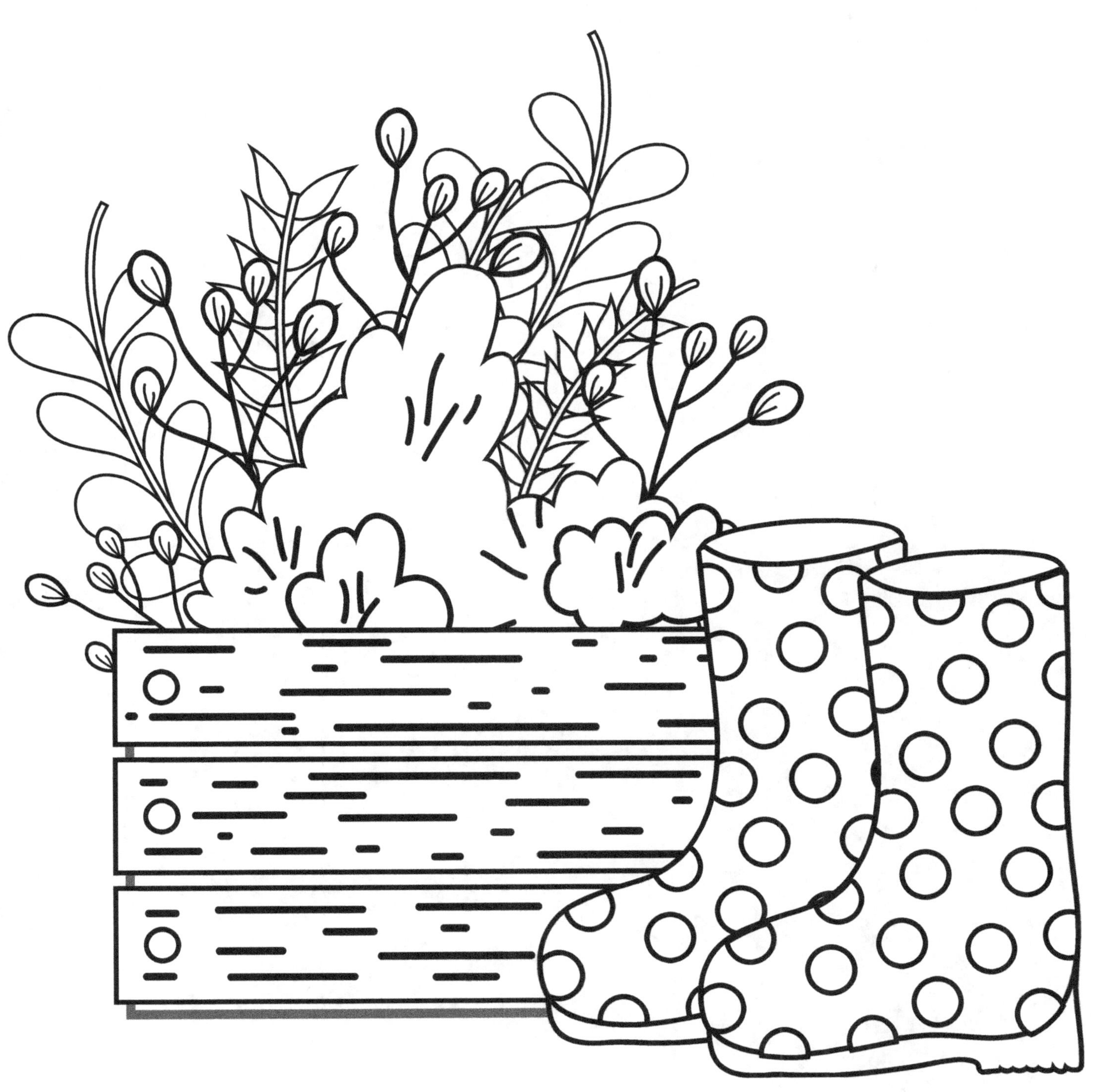

COLORING BOOK

by Little Mary

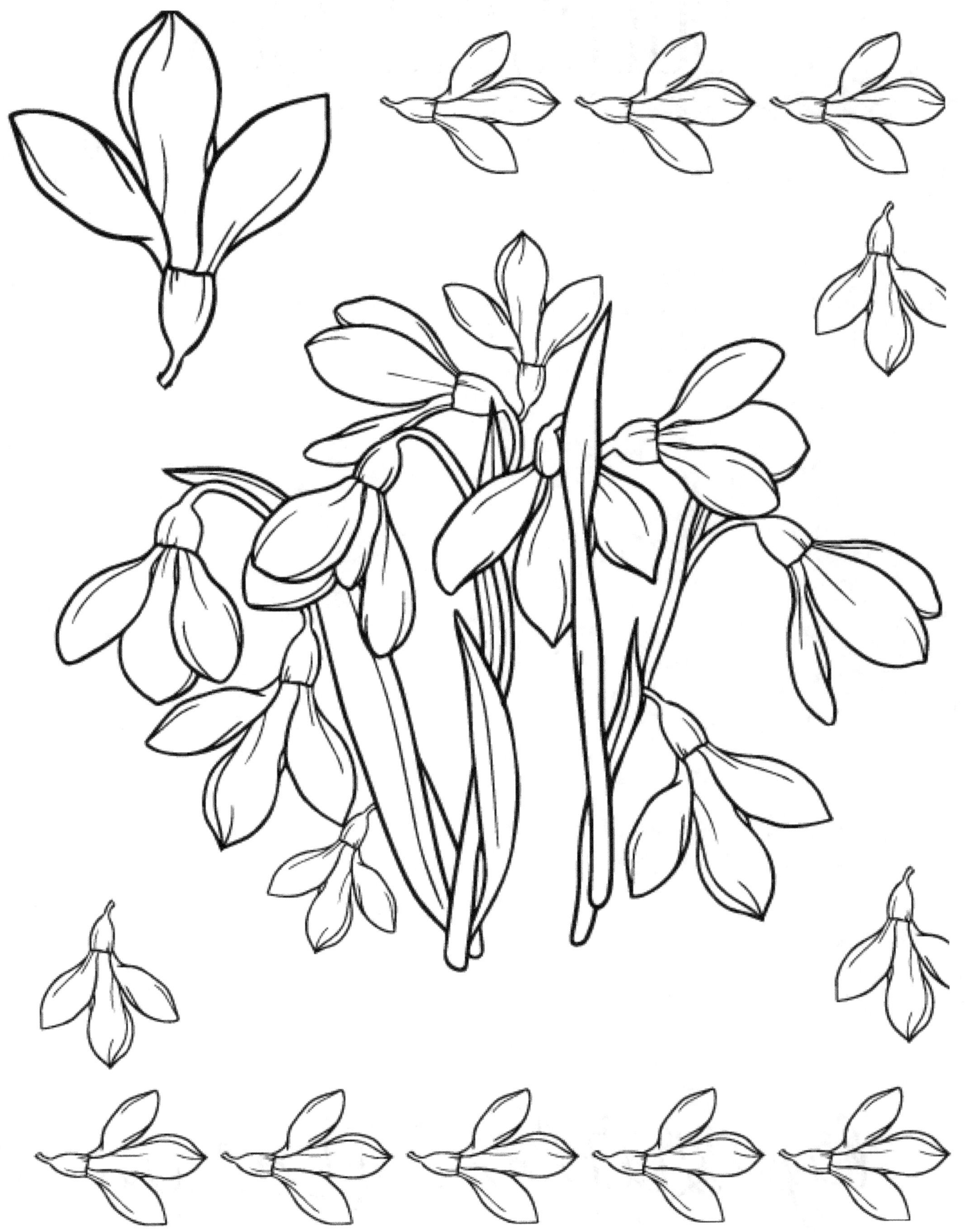

COLORING BOOK

by Little Mary

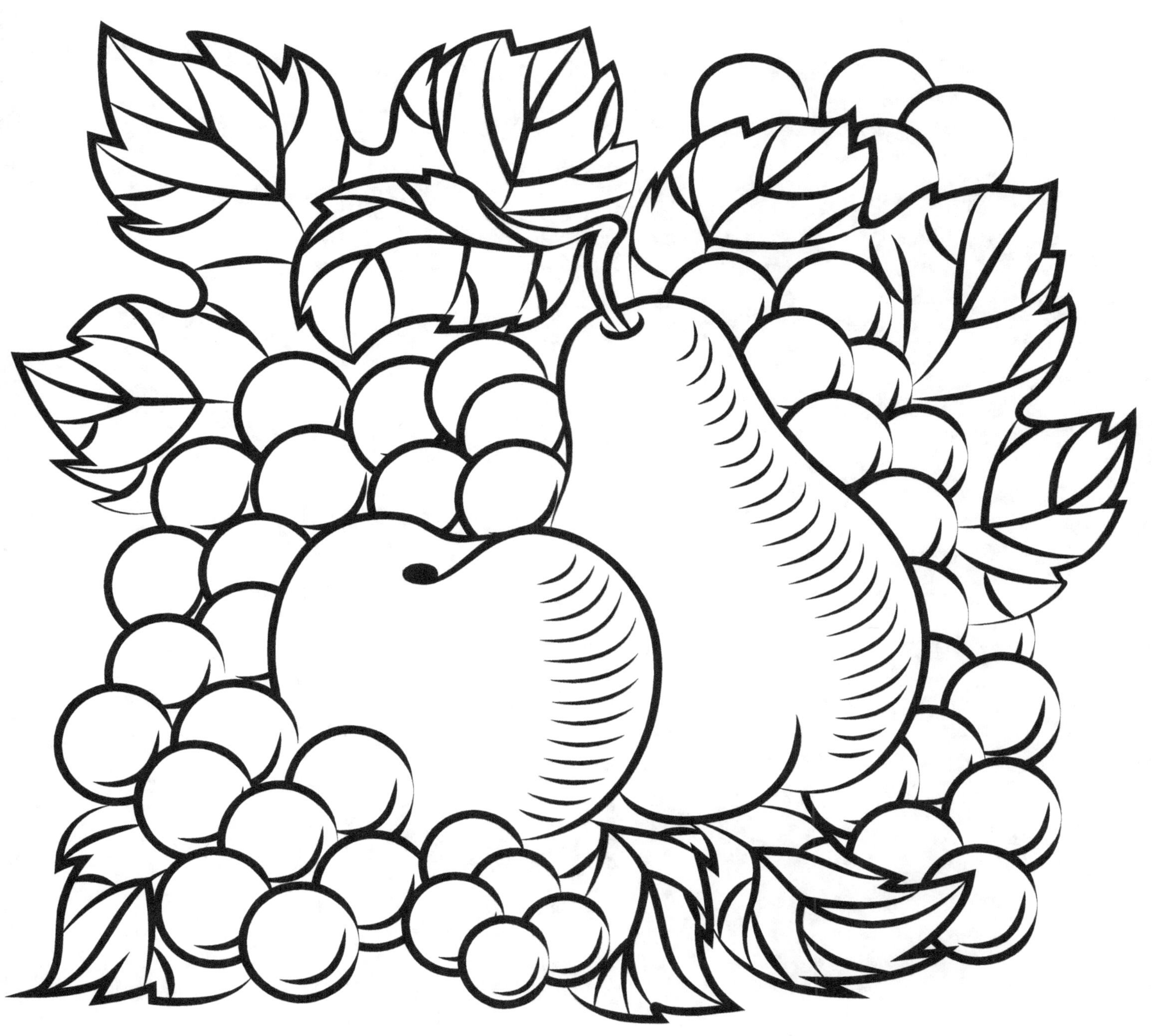

COLORING BOOK

by Little Mary

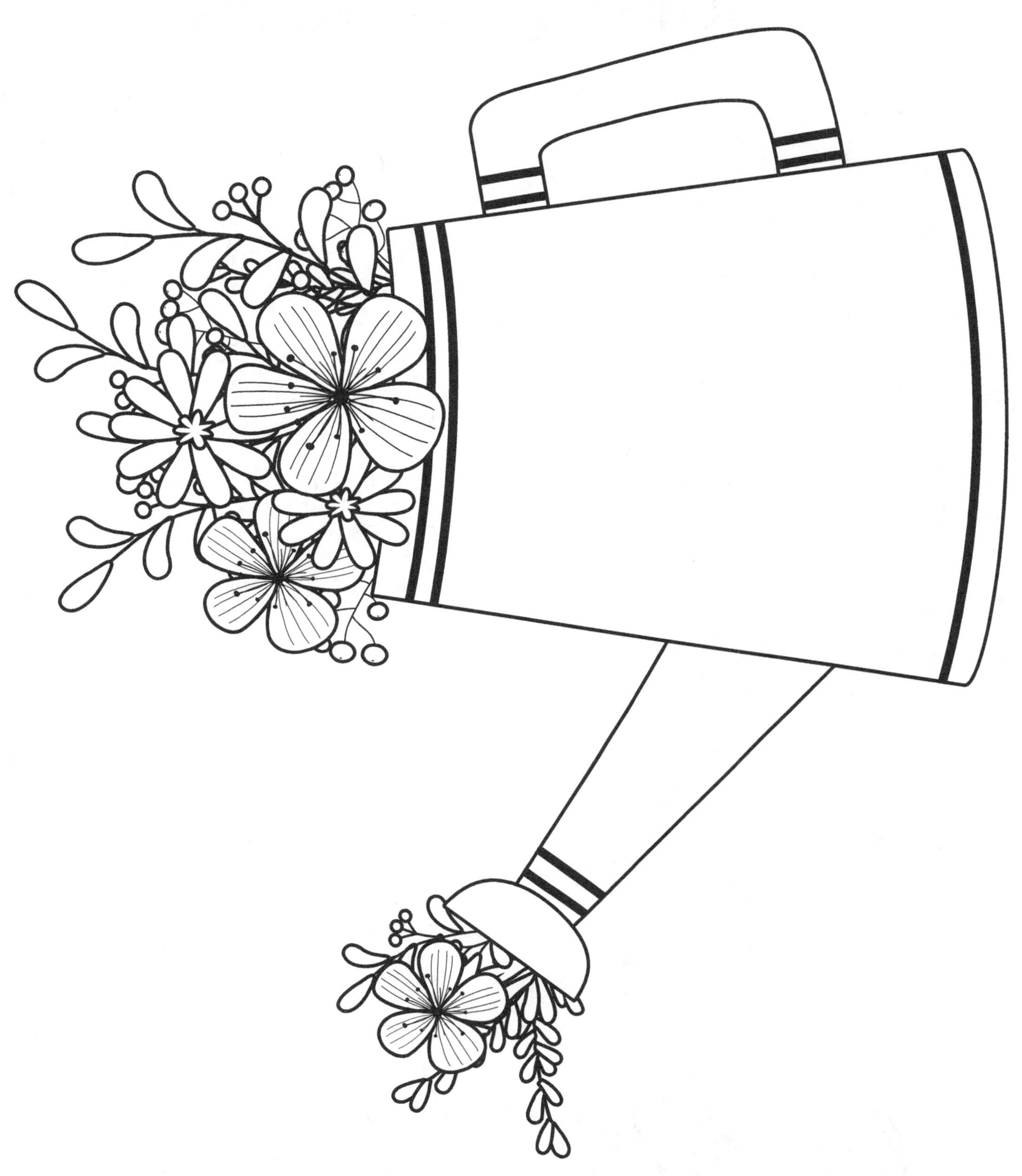

COLORING BOOK

by Little Mary

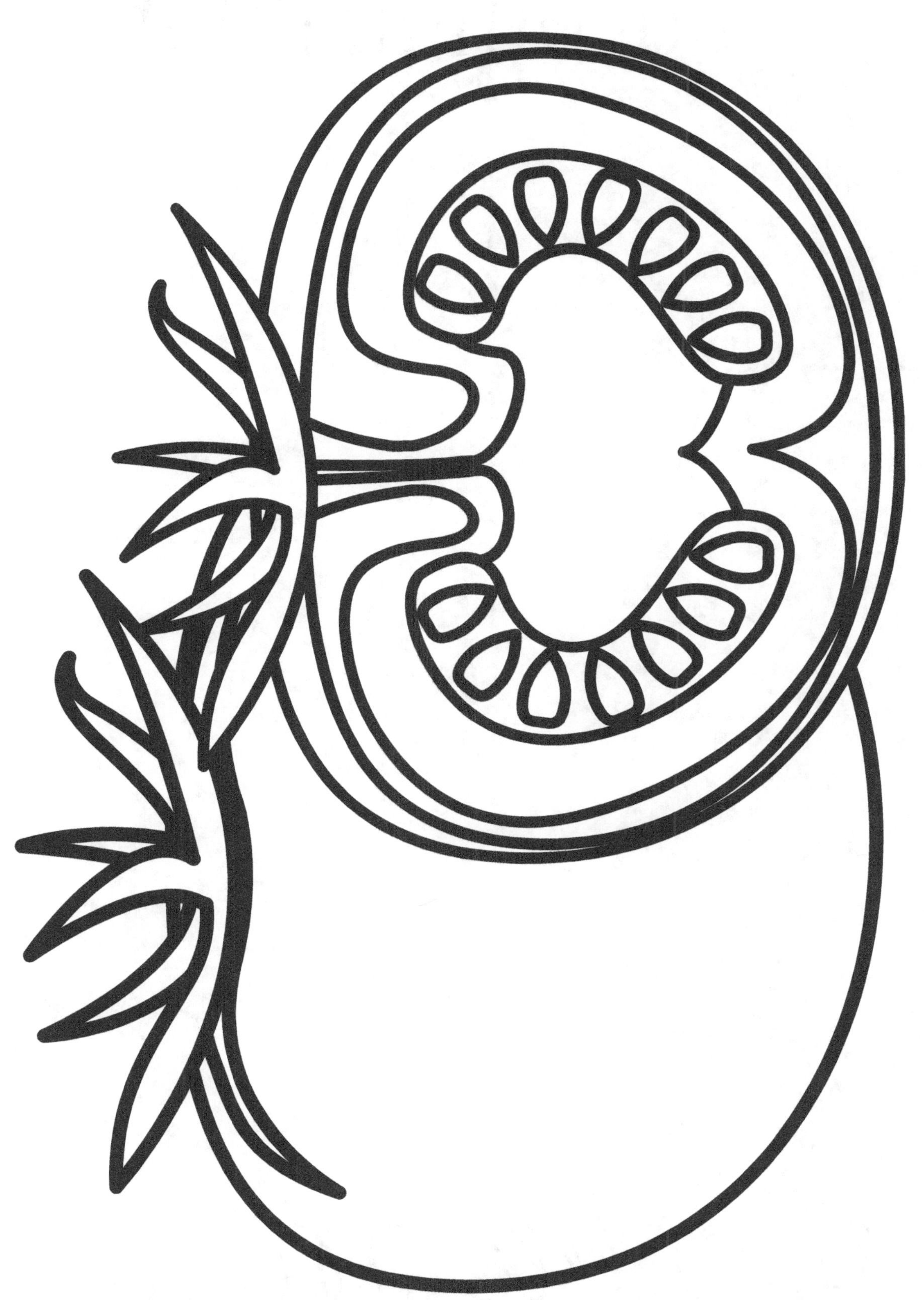

COLORING BOOK

by Little Mary

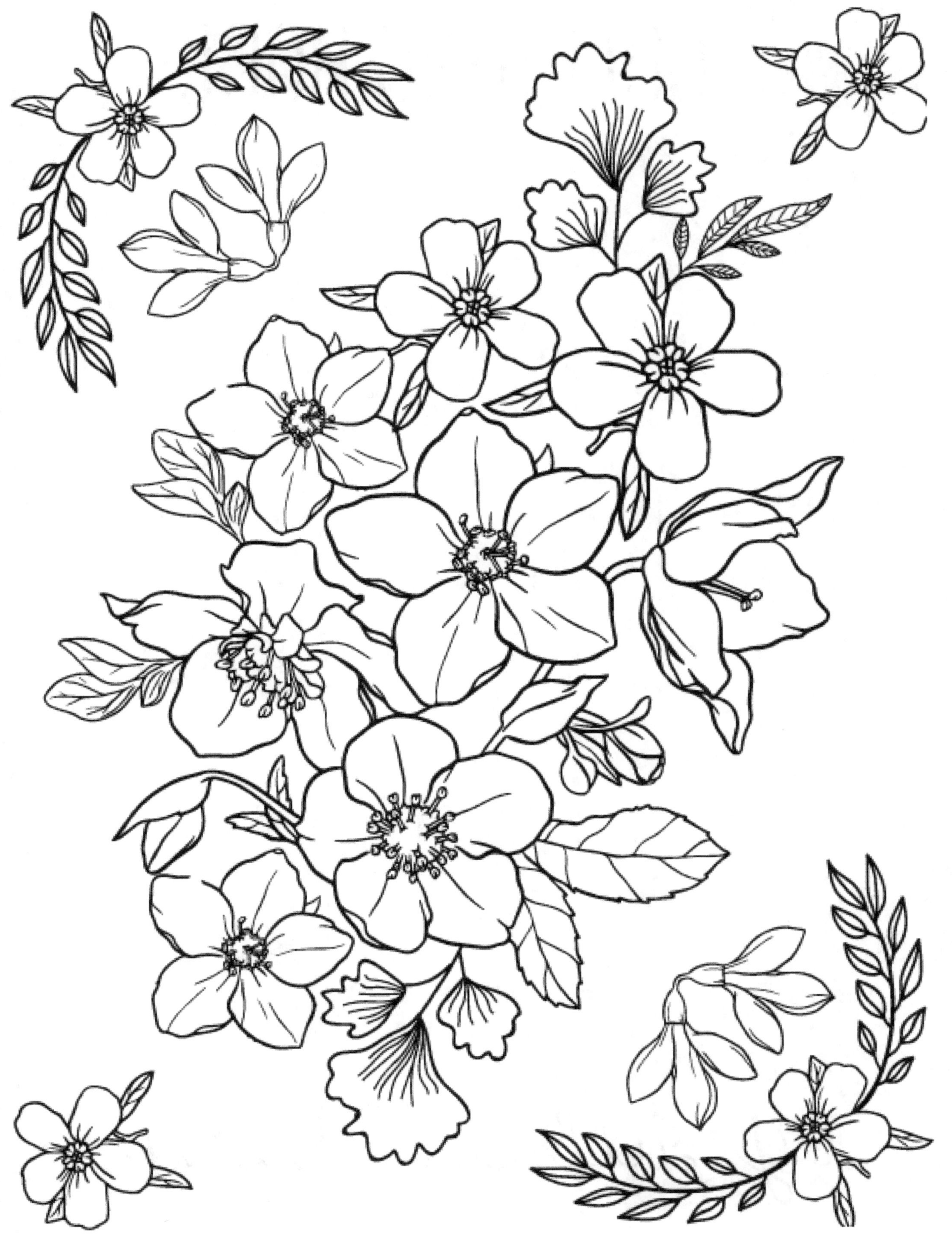

COLORING BOOK

by Little Mary

COLORING BOOK

by Little Mary

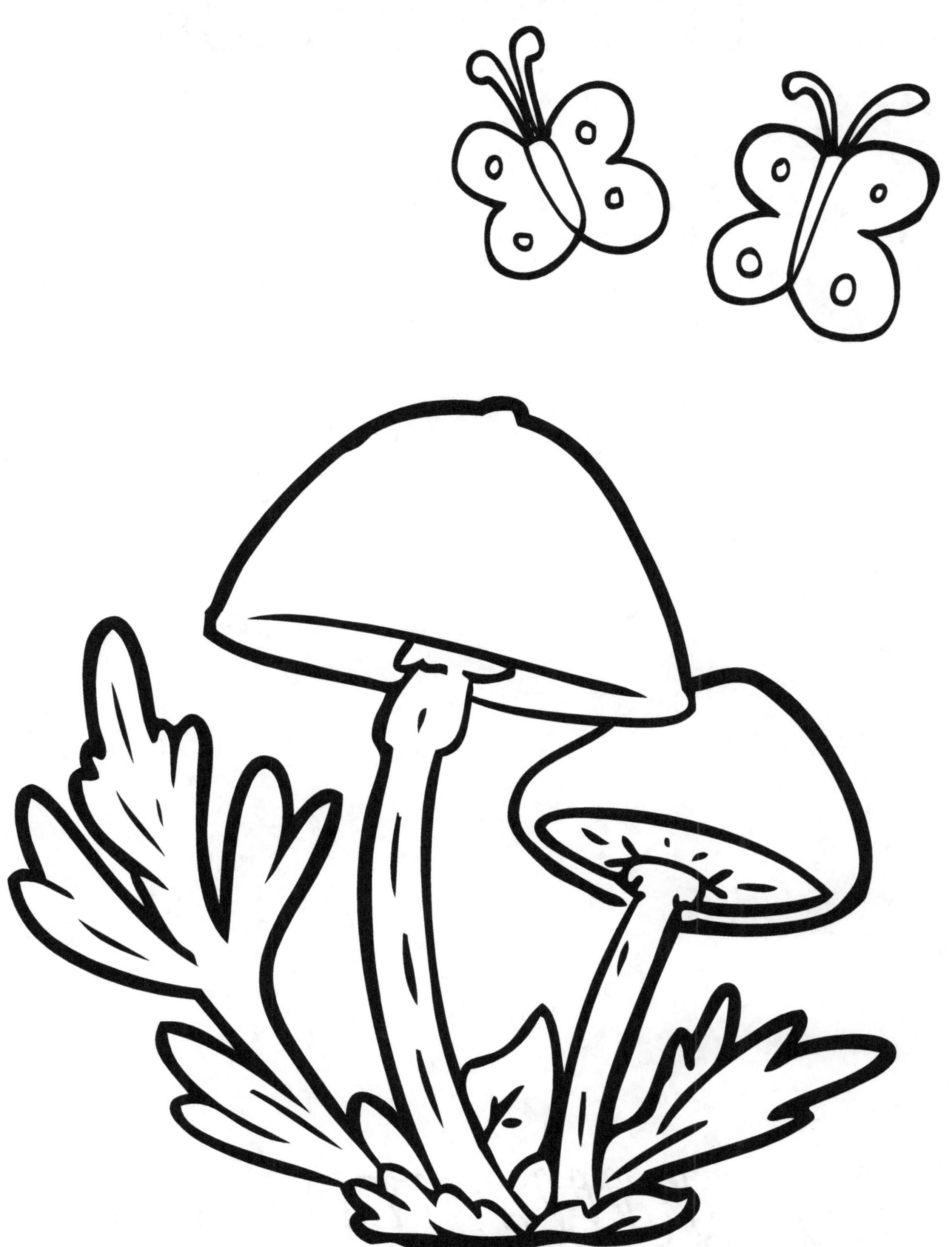

COLORING BOOK

by Little Mary

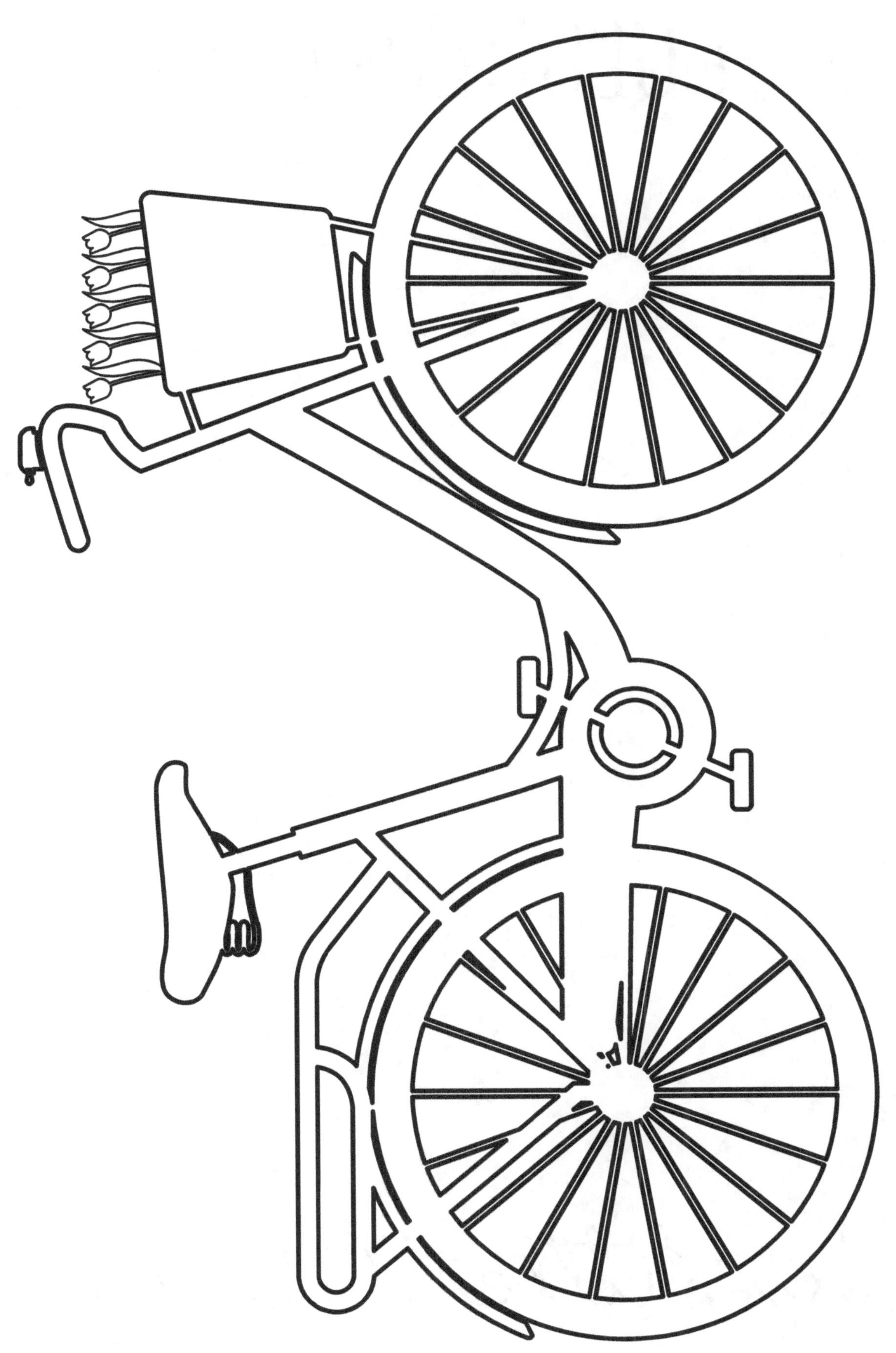

COLORING BOOK

by Little Mary

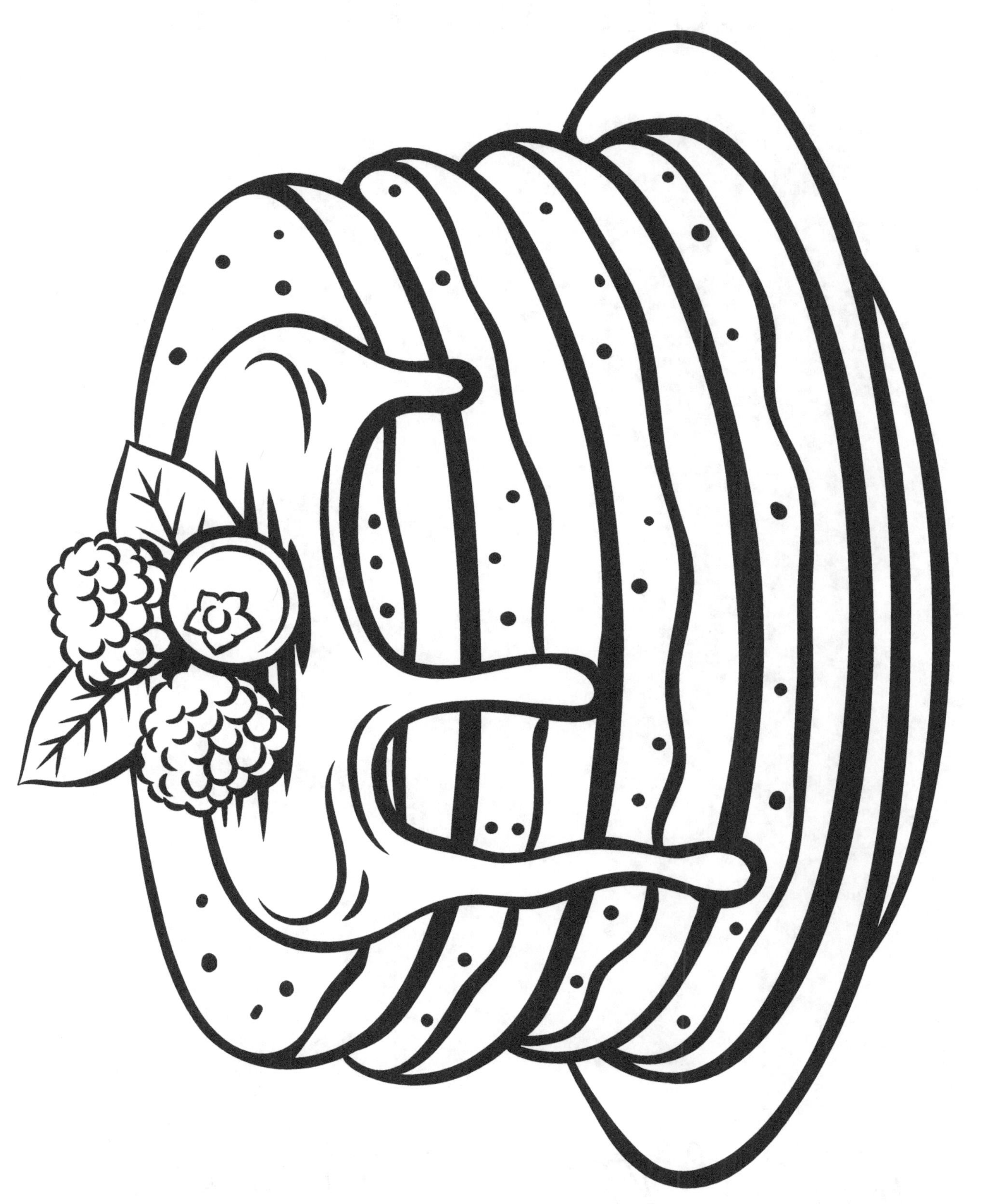

COLORING BOOK

by Little Mary

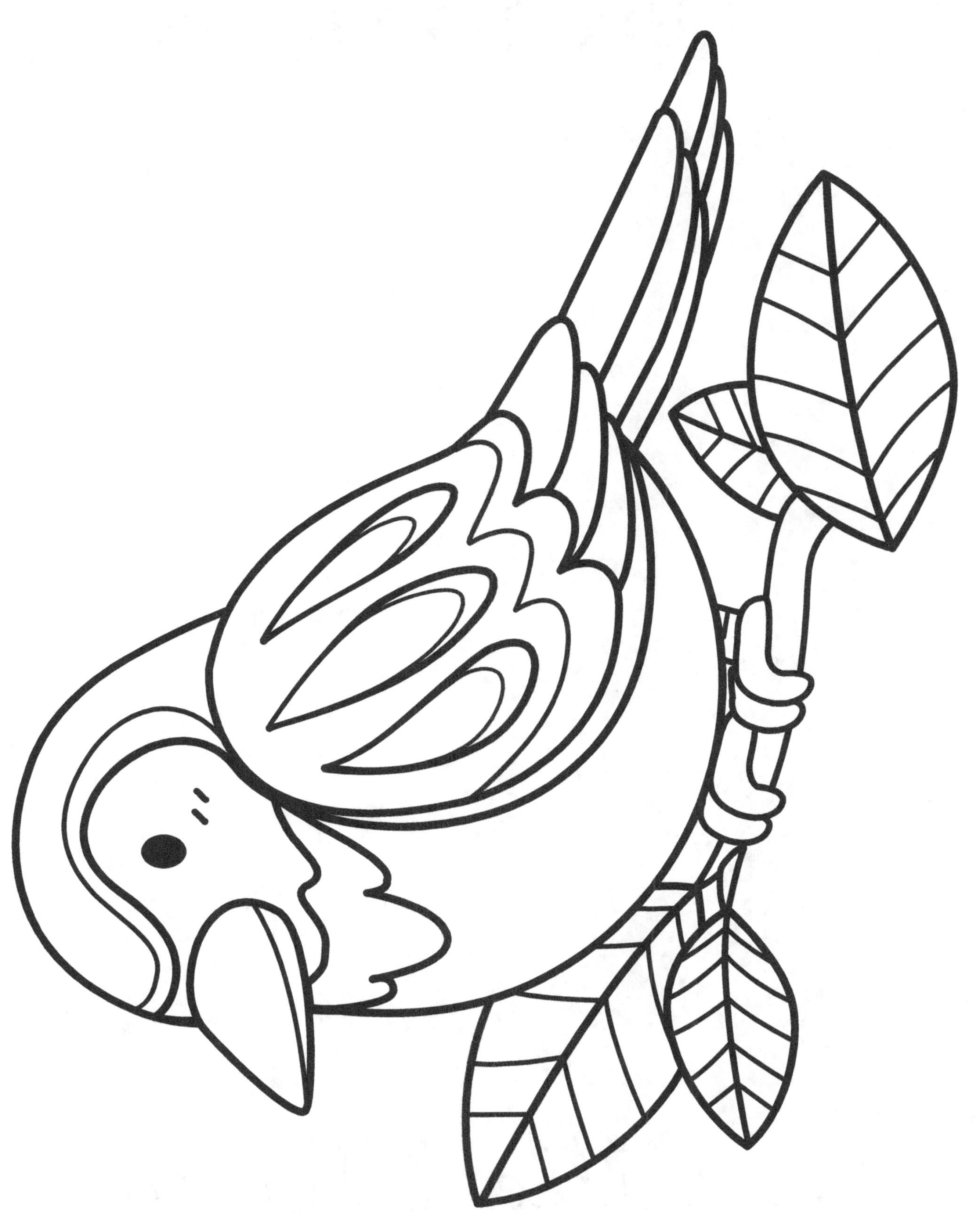

COLORING BOOK

by Little Mary

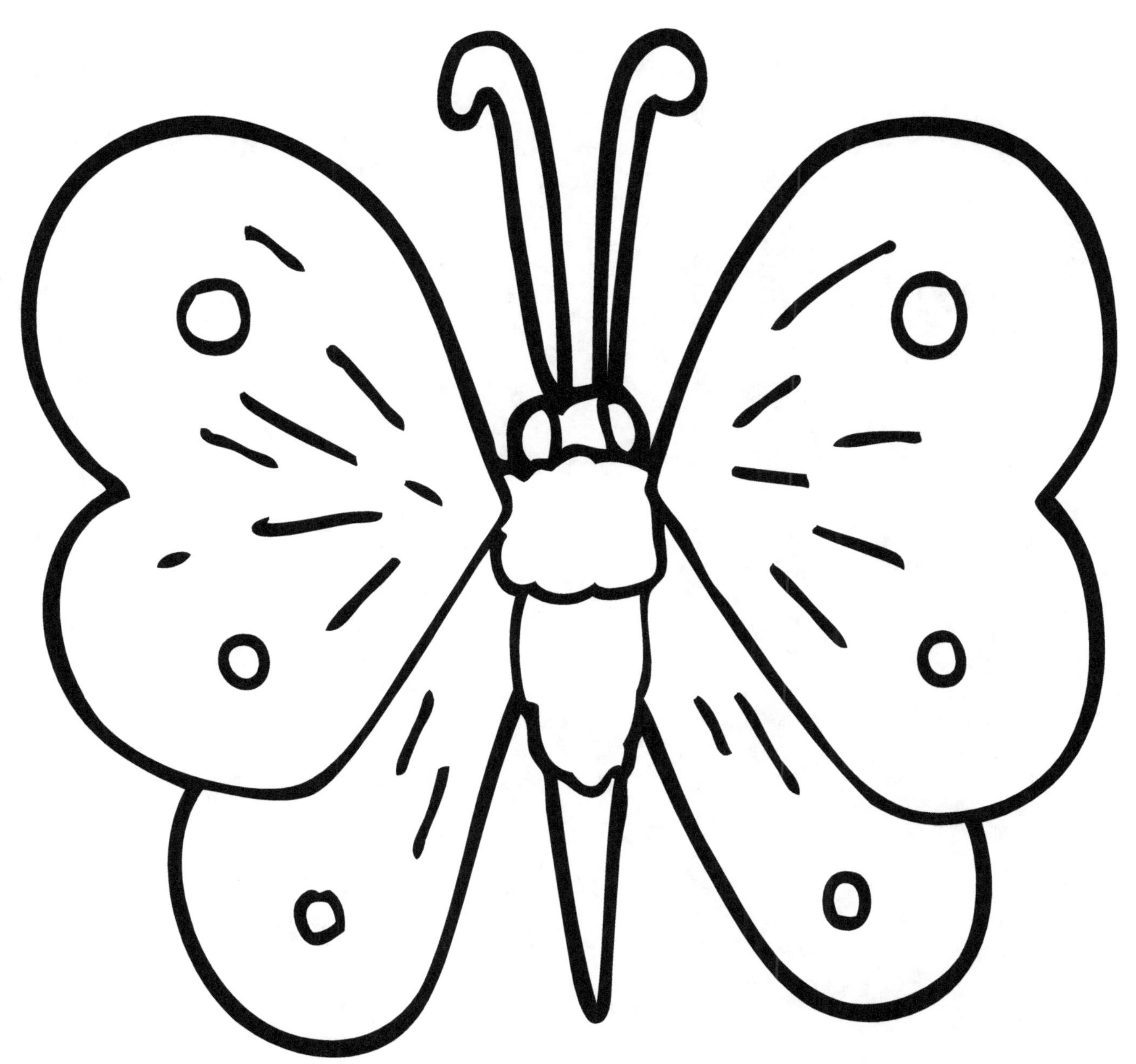

COLORING BOOK

by Little Mary

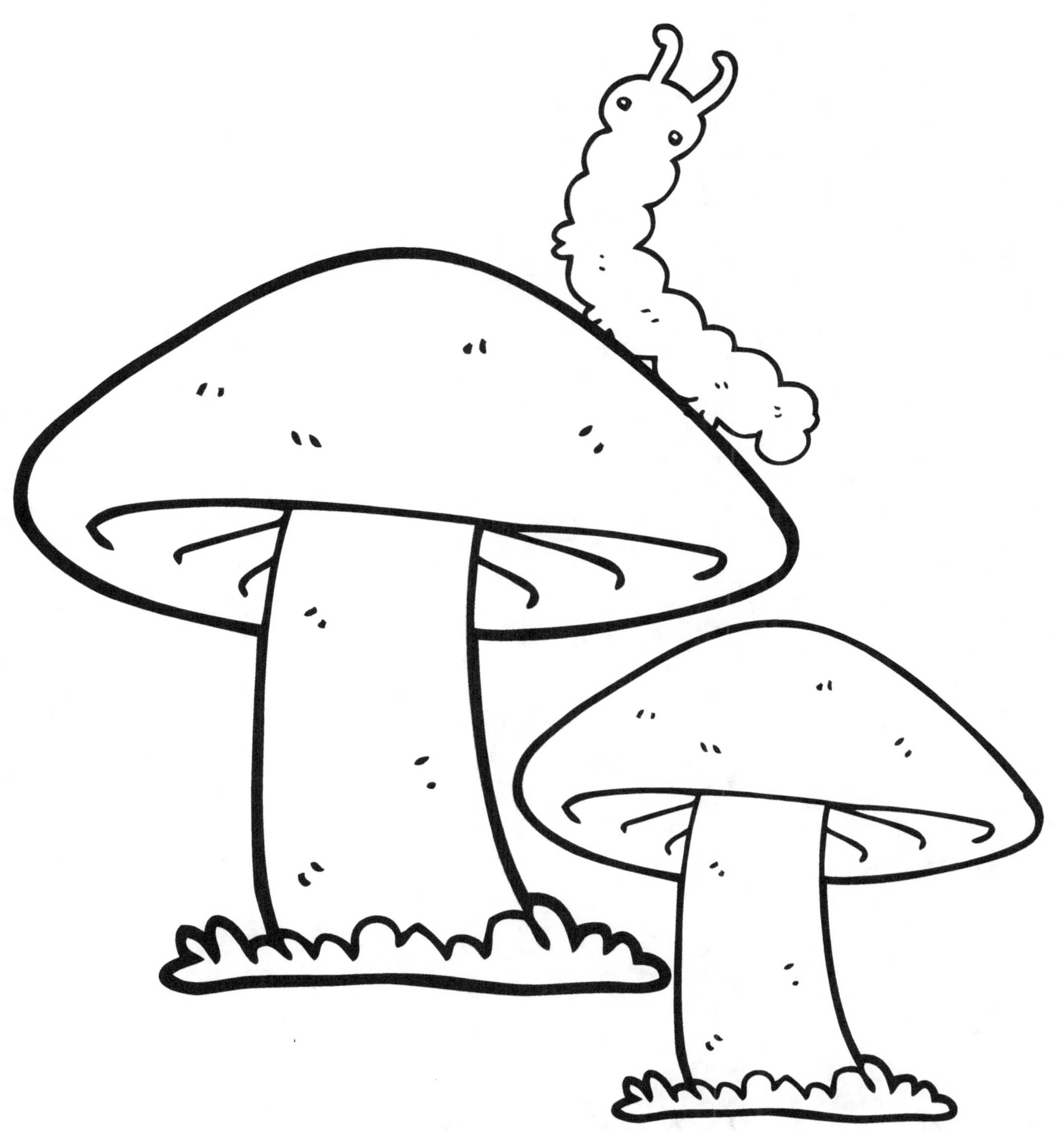

COLORING BOOK

by Little Mary

www.ingramcontent.com/pod-product-compliance
Lightning Source LLC
Chambersburg PA
CBHW081239250726
48654CB00012B/1394